CPC Exam Stud

Certified Professional Coder (CPC®) Exam Study Guide 2020 Edition

Copyright © Medical Coding Pro
All rights reserved.

ISBN: 9781655665462

DEDICATION

To the hard working students preparing for the medical coding certification exam. Your work ethic and dedication to the medical coding industry will ensure its health and competency for years to come!

Copyright Medical Coding Pro
Published by: IPC Marketing LLC
PO Box 3824
Youngstown, Ohio 44513

ALL RIGHTS RESERVED. No part of this book may be reproduced or transmitted in any form whatsoever, electronic, or mechanical, including photocopying, recording, or by any informational storage or retrieval system without the expressed written, dated and signed permission from the author.

DISCLAIMER AND/OR LEGAL NOTICES:

The information presented herein represents the view of the author as of the date of publication. The book is for informational purposes only.

While every attempt has been made to verify the information provided in this book, neither the author nor his affiliates/partners assume any responsibility for errors, inaccuracies or omissions or for any damages related to use or misuse of the information provided in the book.

Any slights of people or organizations are unintentional. If advice concerning medical or related matters is needed, the services of a fully qualified professional should be sought. Any reference to any person or business whether living or dead is purely coincidental.

SAVE $50! Use Coupon Code "SAVE50"

The Medical Coding Certification Prep Course

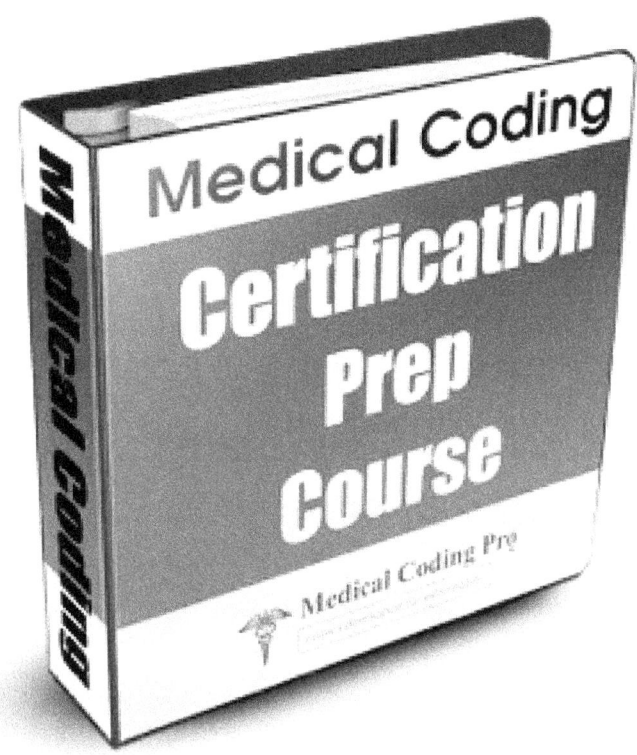

The Medical Coding Certification Prep Course is a web based, self paced, course with over 100 hours of study material. It includes over 700 practice exam questions and answers, 120 Operative Reports, 1,200 terms defined plus current and previous year CPT codes. The course also includes a complete ICD-10 video instruction module, course workbook and one year online access. Professional AAPC approved CPC, COC instructor available to answer questions and give guidance.

For more information go to:

www.MedicalCodingPro.com/medical-coding-certification-prep-course

Quick Start Guide 5

Medical Coding Exam Strategy 6

Overview 16

CPC Mock Exam - 150 Questions 18

CPC Mock Exam - Answers and Rationale 71

Secrets To Reducing Exam Stress 92

Common Anatomical Terminology 119

Medical Terminology Prefix, Root, and Suffixes 124

Notes 137

Scoring Sheets 139

Resources 163

Quick Start Guide

Start by reviewing everything included inside the study guide. Contents include the following:

1) Medical Coding Exam Strategy
2) Overview
3) Mock Exam Questions, Answers, and Rationale
4) Secrets To Reducing Exam Stress
5) Common Anatomical Terminology
6) Medical Terminology Prefixes, Roots, and Suffixes
7) Notes
8) Scoring Sheets
9) Resources

These resource used properly will give you a good base to prepare for the certification exam

If you have any questions please email contact us at support@medicalcodingpro.com.

Thank you for your business!

Medical Coding Exam Strategy

One of the first things we should discuss is what "The Strategy" is and what it isn't.

What it is:

A simple, yet powerful, method for increasing your chances of passing the Medical Coding Certification Exam. Many people have told us that time management was their biggest obstacle in passing the exam. This is what "The Strategy" addresses. It is a road map to pass the exam. It has very little to do with coding knowledge and everything to do with your approach.

What it isn't:

A long, drawn out, hard to follow maze with do's and don'ts reviewing the material that was covered in class. We assume that you know the material, otherwise, it doesn't matter what we teach you the odds are against you.

Why it is important: The reality is many people do not pass the exam the first time. This becomes a costly proposition and one that wasn't bargained for because the next step is an exam retake. The cost: $300. Some even go further and sign up for a three day "boot camp". The cost: about $1200.

Between a rock and a hard place

In this very typical example you passed the Medical Coding class with flying colors but the major hospitals and doctor offices all want a certified medical coder. Why, because it increases their output, makes them more money, and limits their liability for mistakes. So now you're stuck. You have to get certified, but at what cost? It all depends how many times you have to take the certification exam. Follow the steps outlined in "The Strategy" and your next exam could reward you with a certification.

Start by reviewing common mistakes

Some of the most common mistakes made while taking the exam are what we like to call "time wasters". The most important factor to succeeding is time management. You only have 5 hours and 40 minutes to complete the exam (including breaks) and it consists of 150 questions so every minute counts.

The time breakdown goes like this: Exam Time (without breaks) 5 hours 40 minutes or 340 minutes. Exam length: 150 Questions. The easy math is two minute per question. What can we eliminate to save time?

Things Not To Do

1) Answer each question in numerical order.
2) Take too much time on difficult questions first.
3) Read the doctors chart before reading the detail of the question.
4) Not highlighting questions "passed" in the first round

Time Waster #1:

Answering each question in numerical order

If you answer each question in numerical order you will never finish the exam! This is one of the most common mistakes made. If you start out answering the first several questions just fine and then ten questions into the exam you come to a one that you have trouble with, what then? This is a "time burner" and one you can not get hung up on. We will review why this is more important later in "The Strategy".

The Exam is five hours and forty minutes and 150 questions... an average of two minutes per question. The key is to redistribute your time.

Time Waster #2:

Taking too much time on difficult questions the first time through the exam

"The Strategy" is based on a "two pass" system. The first pass is designed to answer the easy questions and highlight the more difficult ones. These will be addressed on the second pass. A good rule of thumb is if you can't answer it in a minute and a half, move on! If you continue to work on these questions you run the risk of not completing the exam or having to rush through the more difficult questions at the end.

Time Waster #3:

Reading the doctors chart before reading the detail of the question

If you get caught in this "time waster" it will rob you of valuable minutes. Always read the question completely before reading the doctors chart. You may be able to eliminate much of the chart because the question is requesting limited information or specific detail.

Time waster #4:

Not highlighting the more difficult questions for the second "pass"

Be prepared. Have a game plan and stick to it. Make sure that you highlight the more difficult questions that you are going to "pass" on in the first round of the exam. If you make the mistake of not highlighting these questions, you will lose valuable minutes trying to search for them in the second round.

Your goal is to answer the easier questions in a minute and a half maximum! Out of 150 questions, let's assume you can answer 60%, or 90 questions, on the first pass averaging 1 minutes per question. That is a total of 135 minutes to answer the first 90 questions. Again, this is an average. That leaves you with 165 minutes to answer the remaining 60 questions. That comes out to 2 minutes per question on the second pass! Now you can be more deliberate with the remaining, more difficult, questions to make sure you answer them correctly.

The "time wasters" have to be minimized or eliminated for you to be successful. Every minute you can save on looking up codes or moving more difficult questions to the second pass the closer you are to your certification.

"Time Wasters" have to be avoided at all costs. Implement a "two pass" system and watch your results increase substantially!

Now let's take an in depth look at the keys that will make all the difference in your exam experience. These are "The Strategy" and "The "Keys" to passing the Medical Coding Certification Exam! These are not difficult, complex strategies. These are straight forward, simple strategies that are easy to implement and highly effective. Follow each step and you will be well on your way to certification.

The Exam Strategy:

1) The basic element of the strategy is making two passes through the exam. The first pass is to answer the questions you can complete in 1 . minute or less. This should be about 60% of the questions. If you can not answer a question in that time, highlight it (mark it for the second pass) and move on! That creates 2 minutes for the remaining 40% which you have identified as more difficult. This should leave you plenty of time on the more difficult questions and improve your overall score.

2) Answer the easier questions in each section on the first pass. You have to answer 70% of the questions or better correctly to pass so answering the easier questions in each section will form a good base of correctly answered questions in all sections thus improving your chances of passing.

3) Identify the first three numbers of the code first. This will help you eliminate answers instantly and narrow your choices for the correct answer. This is a big "time saver". Practice this on your mock practice exam.

4) Read each question before reading the entire doctors chart. Another big "time saver"! Don't waste valuable time reading the entire doctors chart before reading the question. Read the entire question first to find out the specific information the question is requesting.

5) Highlight Procedures one color, Diagnosis another color and Modifiers a third color for quick reference (again, a big time saver!)

The Keys to Success:

Key #1: Study and Preparation.

Don't let anyone fool you into thinking that you don't have to study. That is not the case. You NEED to study, and study hard! The Exam Strategy assumes that you know all the material. There are no shortcuts and The Exam Strategy will only help you pass if you know the material. So put in the time!

One of the best tools available to practice time management for the exam is the Medical Coding Exam System

(www.MedicalCodingExamSystem.com).

It is course dedicated strictly to time management. This will pay big dividends during the exam. We also highly the Faster Coder (www.fastercoder.com) to improve your speed and accuracy. You will quickly find it is worth its weight in gold.

Key #2: Two Complete Passes through the Exam.

During the exam you will be making TWO passes through the entire exam. Let me repeat this because it is at the heart of what we are trying to accomplish. During the exam you will be going through the entire exam twice! The first pass is to answer the easier questions and the second pass is to answer the more difficult ones. Many people do not pass the exam because they get caught up on a few difficult questions and end up not completing the entire exam. You must follow this key element as it is your key to success.

Key #3: Answer The First Pass Questions in 1 1/2 Minutes or Less.

Start the exam by making a first pass. During the first pass answer all the questions that you can complete in a reasonable amount of time (1 1/2 minutes). If you can't answer the question in 1 1/2 minutes highlight it and move on!

Key #4: Highlight All Unanswered Questions in First Pass

If you cannot answer a question within 1 1/2 minutes of the first pass, highlight the unanswered questions in yellow for easy reference during the second pass! Do not forget to highlight them as every second counts and this could be a big time saver!

Key #5: Answer the More Difficult Questions during Second Pass

You should complete the first pass in 135 minutes or less. This will establish a good base of answered questions and leave you with 165 minutes or more to go back and answer the highlighted questions.

Key #6: Do Not Answer the Questions in Order, You Will Fail!

If you take your time and answer the first 120 questions perfect but run out of time and have to guess on the remaining 30 questions, YOU WILL NOT PASS. You must answer 105 questions correctly to pass the exam. (This has been revised to require a 70% pass rating on all questions combined)!

Key #7: Identify the First Three Numbers of the Code

Another good "time saver" is to identify the first three numbers of the code, turn to that page, then go to the sub code numbers.

Key #8: You Can Miss a Certain Percentage in each Section

You can miss a certain percentage in each section and still pass the exam. Your goal is to get enough right to pass. Making two complete passes through the exam will ensures that you are, at minimum, answering the easy questions in each section first. This alone will increase your chances of passing because you will have a base of questions answered in each section. Typically, the last section is rushed through. This will eliminate this hurdle.

Key #9: Read Each Question before Reading the Doctors Chart

Go over each question before you read the doctors chart. This will tell you exactly what you are looking for. You may not need to read the entire chart because the question only references a specific section. This will save you precious time.

Key #10: Highlight Procedures, Diagnosis, and Modifiers

Highlight the patient's treatment/s in different colors for easy reference. I recommend using these colors: Yellow for Procedures, Blue for Diagnosis, and Pink for Modifiers.

Key #11: You Must Answer 70% correctly to pass the exam

You must keep moving! Leave the tough questions and move on. Ask around to anyone who did not pass the exam the first time (or more) and see what they say. It's all about time management and using the right tips and techniques. So to that end, if you do not follow any other advice, follow this! Do the easiest questions first.

Bonus Tips:

1) Eliminate any answers that begin with an E-Code instantly! Cross it out... this will reduce your selection of answers.

2) Code injections with an administration charge.

3) Supervision and Interpretation components require physician supervision. In radiology procedures this means the radiologist has participated.

4) Know the difference between modifier 26 and modifier TC from your HCPCS II book.

5) Diabetes mellitus – etiology code first then the manifestation code.

6) Trauma accident- always code the most severe injury first

7) Tab all your books including CPT, HCPCS Level II, ICD-10-CM, for quick reference.

8) Code burns on the depth of the burn (1st, 2nd, or 3rd degree). Burns are classified to the extent of the body surface involved. When coding burns of multiple sites, assign separate codes for each burn site. Also burns of the same local site (three-character category level, T20-T28), but of different degrees should be coded to the highest degree documented.

9) Multiple fractures, code by site and sequence by severity.

10) If the same bone is fractured or dislocated, code the fracture only.

11) If the question doesn't state open or closed fracture, code as a closed fracture.

12) Late effects (now called "sequela); is a residual of previous illness or injury. Code the residual and then the cause. Reference "late" in the index.

13) Sequence symptoms first if no diagnosis.

14) Study Medicare A, B, C, D

15) Understand modifier 62 co-surgeons (look on exam for surgeon A and B)

16) ***KEEP MOVING, KEEP MOVING, AND KEEP MOVING!***

Overview

Certified Professional Coder (CPC®)

The CPC® Exam

- 150 multiple-choice questions (proctored)
- 5 hours and 40 minutes to finish the exam
- 1 free retake
- $425 ($325 AAPC Students)
- Open code book (manuals)

The CPC examination consists of questions regarding the correct application of CPT®, HCPCS Level II procedure and supply codes and ICD-10-CM diagnosis codes used for coding and billing professional medical services to insurance companies. Examinees must also demonstrate knowledge on proper modifier use, coding guidelines and regulatory rules.

The CPC exam thoroughly covers: 10,000 Series CPT, 20,000 Series CPT, 30,000 Series CPT, 40,000 Series CPT, 50,000 Series CPT, 60,000 Series CPT, Evaluation and Management, Anesthesia, Radiology, Laboratory and Pathology, Medicine, Medical Terminology, Anatomy, ICD-10-CM/ Diagnosis, HCPCS Level II, Coding Guidelines, and Compliance and Regulatory.

Mock Practice Exam Questions & Answers

The following is a Medical Coding Pro Mock Exam. You may not use any outside materials for this exam other than the manuals referenced by the American Academy of Professional Coders (AAPC).

The code research program we use and recommend is Find A Code. You can locate it at: www.findacode.com?pc=MEDCOPRO.

To pass the certification exam you must manage your time carefully. If after going through this practice you determine that time management is a skill you may need additional assistance with, the Medical Coding Exam System (www.MedicalCodingExamSystem.com) is an excellent resource for additional support.

If you want additional resources to prepare for the certification exam we highly recommend FasterCoder.com (www.FasterCoder.com).

CPC Mock Exam - 150 Questions

Section 1: Surgery and Modifiers:

10,000 Series 10 Questions

1. A new patient presents to the urgent care center with a laceration to the left elbow that happened 10 days ago and was not treated. An infected gaping wound was found, with resulting cellulitis to the forearm and upper left arm. Extensive irrigation and debridement using sterile water were performed but closure was not attempted pending resolution of the infection. Culture of the wound revealed streptococcus. The patient received 1,200,000 units of Bicillin CR IM and is to return in 3 days to follow up. The history and physical examination were problem focused.

a. S51.012A, L03.114, B95.5, 99201, 96372, J0561 X 12
b. L03.114, B95.5, 96372-LT, J0561 X12
c. S41.009A, B95.5, 99201
d. S51.012A, 99281, 96372, J0561X12

2. 12-year-old female was chasing her friend when she fell through a sliding glass door sustaining three lacerations. Left knee 5.5 cm laceration, involving deep subcutaneous tissue and fascia, was repaired with layered closure using 1% lidocaine anesthetic. Right knee: 7.2 cm laceration was repaired under local anesthetic with a single-layer closure. Right hand: 2.5 cm laceration of the dermis was repaired with simple closure using Dermabond© tissue adhesive.

ASSESSMENT: Wounds of both knees and left hand requiring suture repair.

PLAN: Follow-up in 10 days for suture removal. Call office if any questions or complications. What are the correct ICD-10-CM and CPT procedure codes? Do not code anesthesia administration.

a. S81.012A, S81.011A, S61.411A, W01.110A, Y92.009, 12005
b. S81.012A, S81.011A, S61.411A, 12002-RT, 12032-51-LT, 17999-51-LT
c. S71.009A, 12032, 12002-LT, A4364
d. S81.012A, S81.011A, S61.411A, W01.110A, Y92.099, 12032-LT, 12004-51-RT

3. Excision lesion on left shoulder, 2.5 x 1.0 x .5 cm, including circumferential margins. Excision lesion, skin of right cheek, 1.0 x 1.0 x .5 cm, including margins. Pathology report states that the skin lesion on the left shoulder is a lipoma and the lesion on the right cheek is a squamous cell carcinoma. The physician progress note states that the left shoulder was sutured with a layered closure, and the cheek was repaired with a simple repair. What are the correct code sets?

a. C44.329, D17.22, 11641-RT, 11403-51-LT, 12031-51-LT
b. C44.329, D17.22, 11641-RT, 12031-51-LT
c. C44.329, D17.21, 11641-RT, 12031-51-LT
d. C44.329, 11643-RT, 12031-51-LT

4. OPERATIVE REPORT

POSTOPERATIVE DIAGNOSIS: Full thickness burn wound to anterior left lower leg. Operation: Split- thickness graft, approximately 35 centimeters; preparation of the wound. Procedure: Left lower leg was prepped and draped in the usual sterile fashion. The ulcer, which measured approximately 8 x 4 to 4.5 cm, was debrided sharply with Goulian knife until healthy bleeding was seen. The bleeding was controlled with epinephrine-soaked lap pads. Split-thickness skin graft was harvested from the left lateral buttock area approximately 4.5 to 5 cm x 8 cm at the depth of 14/1000 of an inch. The graft was meshed to 1 to 1.5 fashion and placed over the prepared wound, stabilized with staples and then Xeroform dressings and dry dressings, wrapped with Kerlix and finally immobilized in a posterior splint. The donor site was covered with Xeroform and dry dressings.

What are the correct procedure codes reported by the physician for this procedure performed in the hospital outpatient surgical suite?

a. 15220-LT, 15221-51-LT, 15002-51-LT
b. 15100-LT
c. 14021-LT, 15002-51-LT
d. 15100-LT, 15002-51-LT

5. OUTPATIENT REPORT

POSTOPERATIVE DIAGNOSIS: Basal Cell Carcinoma of the forehead.

PROCEDURE: Excision of basal cell carcinoma with split-thickness skin graft.

The patient was given a local IV sedation and taken to the operating room suite. The face and right thigh were prepped with pHisoHex soap. The cancer was outlined for excision. The cancer measured approximately 2.5 cm in diameter. The forehead was in filtrated with 1% Xylocaine with 1:1,000,000 epinephrine. The cancer was excised and carried down to the frontalis muscle. The area of the excision measured 5 x 4 cm in total. A suture was placed at the 12 o'clock position. The specimen was sent to pathology for frozen section.

Attention was then turned to the skin graft. A pattern of the defect was transferred to the left anterior thigh using a new needle. A local infiltration was performed on the thigh. Using a free-hand knife, a split-thickness skin graft was harvested. The thigh was treated with Tegaderm and a wrap around kerlix and ace wrap. The skin graft was applied and sutured to the forehead defect with running 5-0 plain catgut.

Xeroform with cotton soaked in glycerin was sutured with 4-0 silk. A sterile dressing was applied. The patient tolerated the procedure well with no complication or blood loss.

a. C76.0, 15120
b. C44.319, 15120
c. C44.319, 15120, 11646
d. C76.0, 15002, 15120

6. A skilled nursing home patient with an indwelling Foley catheter is diagnosed with a serious urinary tract infection due to E. coli caused by the catheter. The catheter is removed, and a urine culture and sensitivity is performed. A temporary catheter is placed through the urethra, and aggressive antibiotic therapy is begun in the emergency room of the hospital. Which of the following code sets will be reported by the ER physician? No medical evaluation was performed because the patient was evaluated by her primary care physician via telephone with the nursing home staff, and orders were called into the hospital.

a. N39.0, B96.20, 51701
b. T83.511A, Y84.6, 51703, 99281
c. T83.511A, N39.0, B96.20, Y84.6, 51702
d. N39.0, T83.511A, Y83.8, 51020

7. A five-year-old boy was brought to the ER by a social worker who discovered him alone in spasms, and seizures. The Social Worker relates that the child's older sister told her the boy was bitten on the hand by a raccoon he played with 11 days ago. No treatment was sought for the injury at the time, but the area was inflamed and hot. According to the Social Worker, the mother is a drug addict and often leaves the children unattended, illness actually began 2 days ago with a headache and restlessness and inflammation at the wound site. The child expired due to cardiorespiratory failure before any effective treatment could be administered. CPR was preformed but was not successful. The physician's diagnosis was listed as Rhabdovirus from infected raccoon bite, not treated due to child neglect. Critical care was provided for 60 minutes. Which of the following code sets will be provided?

a. A82.9, S61.429A, W55.51XA, Y07.12, T76.92XA, 99291, 92950
b. B97.89, 99285
c. R09.2, R56.9, R50.9, S61.429A, W55.51XA, Y07.12, 92950
d. A82.9, R56.9, R50.9, 92950

8. A 49-year-old female sustained injuries to the forehead, 1.5 cm. and a 1 cm. wound to the eyebrow when she hit her steering wheel with her head. The closure was layered. Code the service only.

a. 12001
b. 12011
c. 13131
d. 12051

9. The burn patient had a 20 sq cm Biobrane skin graft the upper right leg and a 30 sq cm Biobrane skin graft of the lower left leg.

a. 15271
b. 15271-RT
c. 15271-RT, 15271-LT, 15272-LT
d. 15271-RT, 15271-LT X 2

10. Stacey a 35-year-old female presents for biopsies of both breasts. The biopsies were done using fine-needle aspiration including ultrasound guidance.

a. 19100-50
b. 19101-50
c. 10005-50
d. 10005, 10006

20000 Series

11. Don a 36-year-old male, fell 4 feet off scaffolding and hit his left heel on the bottom rung of the support, fracturing his calcaneal bone in several locations. The surgeon manipulated the bone pieces back in to position and secured the fracture sites with percutaneous fixation.

a. 28456-LT
b. 28415-LT
c. 28405-LT
d. 28406-LT

12. Tracy a 5-year-old female fell down stairs at a daycare. She hit her coccygeal bone and fractured it. The doctor manually manipulated the bone into the proper alignment and told Tracy's mom to have her sit on a rubber ring to alleviate pain.

a. 27200
b. 27202
c. 27510
d. 28445

13. Fred, a 40-year old carpenter at a local college. While working on a window frame from a ladder, the weld on the rung of the metal ladder loosened and he fell backward 8 ft. He landed on his left hip, dislocating it. Under general anesthesia, the Allis maneuver is used to repair the anterior dislocation of the left hip. The pelvis is stabilized and pressure applied to the thigh to reduce the hip and bring it into proper alignment.

a. 27252
b. 27253-LT
c. 27250-LT
d. 27252-LT

14. A 12-year-old female sustained multiple tibial tuberosity fractures of the left knee while playing soccer at her local track meet. The physician extended the left leg and manipulated several fragments back into place. The knee was then aspirated. A long-leg knee brace was then placed on the knee.

a. 27330-LT
b. 27550-LT
c. 27334-LT
d. 27538-LT

15. By manipulation, under general anesthesia a 6-year-old left tarsal's dislocation was reduced. Correct alignment was confirmed by a two-view intraoperative x-rays. A short leg cast was then applied to the left leg. Code only the reduction service.

a. 28545-LT
b. 28545-LT, 29405-LT, 73620
c. 28545-LT, 29405-LT-51
d. 28540-LT, 73620

16. Dr. Devine applied a cranial halo to Gary to stabilize the cervical spine in preparation for x-rays and subsequent surgery. The scalp was sterilized and local anesthesia injected over the pin insertion sites. Posterior and anterior cranial pins are inserted and the halo device attached.

a. 20664
b. 20664, 96372
c. 20661
d. 20661, 96372

17. Charley was playing in the backyard when his sister fired a pellet gun at his left leg and hit him from close range. The pellet penetrated the skin and lodged in the muscle underlying the area. The doctor removed the pellet without complication or incident. Code the procedure only.

a. 10121-LT
b. 20520-LT
c. 20525-LT
d. 10120-LT

18. Steve presents with a deep, old hematoma on his right shoulder. After examination of the shoulder area, the doctor decides that the hematoma needs to be incised and drained.

a. 10160-RT
b. 23030-RT
c. 10140-RT
d. 10060-RT

19. The surgeon performed an arthrodesis, including a laminectomy of the L1 and L2 segments. Approach was posterior with a posterior interbody technique.

a. 22630, 22632
b. 22633 X 2
c. 22634 X 2
d. 22633, 22634

20. Brandon comes into the orthopedic department today with his father after falling from the top bunk bed, where he and his sister were playing. He is having pain in his left lower leg and is unable to bear weight on it. Brandon is taken to the x-ray department. After the physician talks with the radiologist regarding the diagnosis of sprained ankle, the physician decides to apply a short leg cast, designed for walking, just below Brandon's knee to his toes.

a. 29405-LT, S93.402A, W06.XXXA, Y92.013
b. 29425-LT, S93.402A, W06.XXXA, Y92.013
c. 29515-LT, S93.402A, W19.XXXA, Y92.013
d. 29405-LT, S93.402A, W06.XXXA

21. A child is seen in the office for a superficial laceration of the right knee. The physician repairs the 3.0 cm. laceration with simple suturing.

a. 12002-RT
b. 13120-RT
c. 12031-RT
d. 12007-50

22. A woman presents to the Emergency Department for a deep 3.5 cm wound of the right arm. A routine cleansing and layer closure was required.

a. 12031-RT
b. 12032-RT
c. 10121-RT
d. 10061-RT

23. Sam is treated for multiple wounds of the right forearm, hand and knee. The physician sutured the following: simple repair, 2.5 cm forearm; intermediate repair, 1.5 cm. hand; 2.0 cm. simple repair, right knee.

a. 12041-RT, 12002-RT
b. 12041-RT, 12002-RT-51
c. 11600-RT, 11420-RT
d. 11400-RT, 11420-51-RT

30000 Series

24. A 69-year-old male is admitted for coronary ASHD. A prior cardiac catheterization showed numerous native vessels to be 70% to 100% blocked. The patient was then taken to the operating room. After opening the chest and separating the rib cage, a coronary artery bypass was performed using five venous grafts and four coronary arterial grafts. Code the graft procedure(s) and the diagnosis:

a. 33514, I25.10
b. 33536, 33517-51, I25.9
c. 33533, 33522, I25.810
d. 33536, 33522, I25.10

25. An arterial catheterization is coded how?

a. 36600
b. 36620
c. 36640
d. 36620, 36625

26. A patient is taken to the operating room for a ruptured spleen. A partial splenectomy and repair of a rupture was done.

a. 38101, S36.032A
b. 38101-58, 38115-51, D73.5
c. 38115, D73.5
d. 38120, S36.032A

27. A 50-year-old patient has a PICC line with a port placed for chemotherapy infusion. Fluoroscopic guidance was used to gain access to check placement.

a. 35656, 77001
b. 36568, 76937
c. 36571, 76937
d. 36571, 77001

28. Code for a transcatheter aortic valve replacement with prosthetic valve via left thoracotomy:

a. 33363-LT
b. 33364-LT
c. 33365-LT
d. 33366-LT

29. For revascularization therapy of the femoral/popliteal territory, how many codes should be used for a combination angioplasty, stent and angioplasty?

a. One
b. Three
c. One but use an Add-On Code for any additional Vessels
d. None of the answers are correct

30. PREOPERATIVE DIAGNOSIS: Deviated septum

PROCEDURE PERFORMED: Septoplasty; Resection of inferior turbinates
The patient was taken to the operating room and placed under general anesthesia. The fracture of the inferior turbinates was first performed to do the septoplasty. Once this was done, the septoplasty was completed and the turbinates were placed back in their original position. The patient was taken to recovery in satisfactory condition. Code the procedure(s) and the diagnosis:

a. 30520, 30140-51, J34.2
b. 30520, 30130, J34.2
c. 30520, 30130-51, J34.2
d. 30520, 30140-51, S02.2XXA

31. The patient is seen at the clinic for chronic sinusitis. It is determined that an endoscopic sinus surgery is scheduled for the next day. The patient arrives for same-day surgery, and the physician performs an endoscopic total ethmoidectomy with an endoscopic maxillary antrostomy with removal of maxillary tissue. Code the procedure(s) and diagnosis.

a. 31255, 31267-51, J32.9
b. 31200, 31225-51, J32.9
c. 31254, 31256-51, J32.9
d. 31255, 31267-51, J01.90

40000 series

32. Gary is admitted to same-day surgery for a laparoscopic cholecystectomy.

a. 47562
b. 47600
c. 47562, 47550
d. 47570

33. Code an excision of a ruptured appendix with generalized peritonitis.

a. 49020
b. 49020, 49060-51
c. 44960
d. 44960-22

34. Code an ERCP with sphincterotomy.

a. 43260
b. 43264
c. 43262
d. 43262, 43273

35. When the physician does not specify the method used to remove a lesion during an endoscopy, what is the appropriate procedure?

a. Assign the removal by snare technique code as a default.
b. Assign the removal by hot biopsy forceps code.
c. Assign the ablation code.
d. Query the physician as to the method used.

36. Excision of parotid tumor or gland or both. Once the patient was under general anesthesia, successfully, Dr White, assisted by Dr. Green, opened the area in which the parotid gland is located. After inspecting the gland, the decision was made to excise the total gland because of the size of the tumor (5 cm.). With careful dissection and preservation of the facial nerve, the parotid gland was removed. The wound was cleaned and closed, and the patient was brought to recovery in satisfactory condition. Report Dr. Green's service.

a. 11426, D49.89
b. 42420-80, D49.89
c. 42410-80, 97597, C07
d. 42426-62, D11.0

37. This 10-year-old girl presents for a tonsillectomy because of chronic tonsillitis and possible adenoidectomy. On inspection the adenoids were found not to be inflamed. Only the tonsillectomy was done. Code the tonsillectomy only.

a. 42825, J35.01
b. 42820, J35.1
c. 42826, 42835-51, J35.03
d. 42830, 42825-51, J35.1

38. Which code would you use to report a rigid proctosigmoidoscopy with guide wire?

a. 45303
b. 45346
c. 52260
d. 45386

39. A 63-year-old male present to Acute Surgical Care for a sigmoidoscopy. The physician inserts a flexible scope into the patient's rectum and determines the rectum is clear of polyps. The scope is advanced to the sigmoid colon, and a total of three polyps are found. Using the snare technique, the polyps are removed. The remainder of the colon is free of polyps. The flexible scope is withdrawn.

a. 44110, C18.9
b. 44111, C18.7
c. 45388, D12.5
d. 45338, D12.5

40. This woman is in for multiple external hemorrhoids. After inspection of the hemorrhoids, the physician decides to excise all the hemorrhoids.

a. 46250, K64.4
b. 46083, K64.0
c. 46615, K64.8
d. 46255, K64.0

50000 series

41. OPERATIVE REPORT DIAGNOSIS: Acute renal insufficiency

PROCEDURE: Renal biopsy

The patient was taken to the operating room for percutaneous needle biopsy of the right and left kidneys.

a. 50200-50
b. 49000-50
c. 50555-50
d. 50542-LT, 50542-RT

42. Code a biopsy of the bladder?

a. 52354
b. 52204
c. 52250
d. 52224

43. OPERATIVE REPORT

DIAGNOSIS: Large bladder neck obstruction

PROCEDURE PERFORMED: Cystoscopy and transsurethral resection of the prostate.

The patient is a 76-year-old male with obstructive symptoms and subsequent urinary retention. The patient underwent the usual spinal anesthetic, was put in the dorsolithotomy position, prepped, and draped in the usual fashion. Cystoscopic visualization showed a marked high-riding bladder. Median lobe enlargement was such that it was difficult even to get the cystoscope over. Inside the bladder, marked trabeculation was noted. No stones were present.

The urethra was well lubricated and dilated. The resectoscopic sheath was passed with the aid of an obturator with some difficulty because of the median lobe. TURP of the median lobe was performed, getting several big loops of tissue, which helped to improve visualization. Anterior resection of the roof was carried out from the bladder neck. Bladder-wall resection was taken from the 10 to 8 o'clock position. This eliminated the rest of the median lobe tissue as well. The patient tolerated the procedure well. Code the procedure(s) performed and the diagnosis.

a. 52450, 52001-51, N32.0
b. 52450, 52000, Q64.31
c. 52450, 52001, Q64.31
d. 52450, 52000-59, N32.0

44. Code reconstruction of the penis for straightening of chordee:

a. 54300
b. 54435
c. 54328
d. 54360

45. New born clamp circumcision

a. 54161
b. 54162
c. 54150
d. 54150-52

46. Sam is a 40-year-old male in for a bilateral vasectomy that will include three postoperative semen examinations.

a. 55250 X 3
b. 52648
c. 55250
d. 52402 X 3

47. Patient is seen for Bartholin's gland abscess. The abscess is incised and drained by the physician

a. 56405
b. 53060
c. 50600
d. 56420

48. A 22-year-old female is seen at the clinic today for a colposcopy. The physician will take multiple biopsies of the cervix uteri.

a. 57455
b. 57461
c. 56821
d. 57420

49. Sara is a 36-year-old female diagnosed with an ectopic pregnancy. The patient was taken to the operating room for treatment of a tubal ectopic pregnancy, abdominal approach.

a. 59121
b. 59120
c. 59150
d. 59130

50. Code a cesarean delivery including the postpartum care.

a. 59622
b. 59400
c. 58611, 59430
d. 59515

51. D&C performed for a woman with dysfunctional bleeding.

a. 58100
b. 58120
c. 59160
d. 57505

52. Incision into abscess of scrotal wall to drain pus.

a. 11004
b. 54700
c. 55100
d. 11006

60000 series

53. OPERATIVE REPORT DIAGNOSIS: Malignant tumor, thyroid

PROCEDURE: Thyroidectomy, total.

The patient was prepped and draped. The neck area was opened. With careful radical dissection of the neck completed, one could visualize the size of the tumor. The decision was made to do a total thyroidectomy. Note: The pathology report later indicated that the tumor was malignant.

a. 60254, C73
b. 60240, C73
c. 60271, C73
d. 60220, C37

54. Report the codes you would use for burr hole(s) to drain an abscess of the brain?

a. 61253
b. 61156
c. 61150
d. 61151

55. In the operating room the doctor repaired an aneurysm of the intracranial artery by balloon catheter.

a. 61710
b. 61697
c. 61698
d. 61700

56. Removal of a foreign body embedded in the eyelid.

a. 67830
b. 67801
c. 67413
d. 67938

57. Karen is a 13-year-old with chronic otitis media. The patient was taken to same-day surgery and placed under general anesthesia. Dr. White performed a bilateral tympanostomy with the insertion of ventilating tubes. The patient tolerated the procedure well.

a. 69421-50, 69433-51, H66.13
b. 69420-50, H66.43
c. 69436-50, H66.93
d. 69436-50, H67.9

58. Karen, a 14-year-old female, is seen today for removal of bilateral ventilating tubes that Dr. White inserted 1 year ago. General anesthesia is used.

a. 69424
b. 69424-50
c. 69436
d. 69424-50-78

59. Revision mastoidectomy resulting in a radical mastoidectomy.

a. 69502
b. 69511
c. 69602
d. 69603

60. Biopsy of the upper left eyelid:

a. 67810, 69990
b. 67801
c. 67700-E1
d. 67810-E1

61. Strabismus correction involving the lateral rectus muscle.

a. 67314
b. 67311
c. 67318
d. 67312

62. Excisional transverse blepharotomy with one-quarter lid margin rotation graft.

a. 67966
b. 67950
c. 67961
d. 67961, 15576

Section 2: E/M; Radiology, Path & Lab, Medicine

Evaluation & Management

63. A 90-year-old patient asks for a second opinion when he was recently diagnosed with bilateral senile cataracts. His regular ophthalmologist has recommended implantation of lenses after surgical removal of the cataracts. The patient presents to the clinic stating that he is concerned about the necessity of the procedure. During the detailed history, the patient states that he has had decreasing vision over the last year or two but has always had excellent vision. He cannot recall a trauma to the eye in the past. The physician conducted a detailed visual examination and confirmed the diagnosis of the patient's ophthalmologist. The medical decision-making was of low complexity.

a. 99252
b. 99241
c. 99203
d. 92002

64. The attending physician requests a confirmatory consultation from an interventional radiologist for a second opinion about a 60-year-old male with abnormal areas within the liver. The recommendation for a CT guided biopsy is requested, which the attending has recommended be performed. During the comprehensive history, the patient reported right upper quadrant pain. His liver enzymes were elevated. Previous CT study revealed multiple low attenuation areas within the liver (infection not tumor). The laboratory studies were creatinine, 0.9; hemoglobin, 9.5; PT and PTT, 13.0/31.5 with an INR of 1.2. The comprehensive physical examination showed that the lungs were clear to auscultation and the heart had regular rate and rhythm. The mental status was oriented times three. Temperature, intermittent low-grade fever, up to 101° Fahrenheit, usually occurs at night. The CT-guided biopsy was considered appropriate for this patient. The medical decision making was of high complexity.

a. 99223
b. 99245
c. 99255
d. 99221

65. A cardiology consultation is requested for a 69-year-old inpatient for recent onset of dyspnea on exertion and chest pain. The comprehensive history reveals that the patient cannot walk three blocks without exhibiting retrosternal squeezing sensation with shortness of breath. She relate that she had the first episode 3 months ago, which she attributed to indigestion. Her medical history is negative for stroke, tuberculosis, cancer, or rheumatic fever but includes seborrheic keratosis and benign positional vertigo. She has no known allergies. A comprehensive physical examination reveals pleasant, elderly female in no apparent distress. She has a blood pressure of 150/70 with a heart rate of 76. Weight is 131 pounds, and she is 5 foot 4 inches. Head and neck reveal JBP less than 5 cm. Normal carotid volume and upstroke without bruit. Chest examination shows clear to auscultation with no rales, crackles, crepitations, or wheezing. Cardiovascular examination reveals a normal PMI without RV lift. Normal S1 and S2 with an S3 without murmur are noted. The medical decision making complexity is high based on the various diagnosis options.

a. 99223
b. 99254
c. 99255
d. 99245

66. A new patient presents to the emergency department with an ankle sprain received when he fell while roller-blading. The patient is in apparent pain, and the ankle has begun to swell. He is unable to flex the ankle. The patient reports that he did strike his head on the sidewalk as a result of the fall. The physician completes an expanded problem focused history and examination. The medical decision making complexity is low.

a. 99232
b. 99282
c. 99202
d. 99284

67. A physician provides a service to a new patient in a custodial care center. The patient is a paraplegic who has pneumonia of moderate severity. The physician performed an expanded problem- focused history and examination. The examination focused on the respiratory and cardiovascular systems, based on the patients' current complaint and past history of tachycardia. The medical decision making was of low complexity.

a. 99236
b. 99325
c. 99342
d. 99308

68. A new patient is admitted to the observation unit of the local hospital after a 10 foot fall from a ladder. The patient hit his head on the side of the garage as he fell into a hedge that somewhat broke his fall. He has significant bruising on the left side of his body and complains of a 5 out of 10 pain under his left arm. The physician completed a comprehensive history and physical examination. It was decided to admit the patient to observation based on some evidence that he may have hit the left side of his head during the fall. The medical decision making is moderately complex. Also code for a subsequent observation, one day, Expanded, Problem-Focused History, Expanded, Problem- Focused Exam and Moderate Medical Decision Making; what is noteworthy about the subsequent day observation codes?

a. 99222, 99223, They are Add-On Codes
b. 99219, 99225, They are Out of Order Codes
c. 99235, 99224, They are Modifier 51 Exempt
d. 99220, 99226, They Do Not Follow E & M Rules of the Three Key Components.

69. An established patient is admitted to the hospital by his attending physician after a car accident in which the patient hit the steering wheel of the automobile with significant enough force to fold the wheel backward. The patient complains of significant pain in the right shoulder. After a detailed history and physical examination, the physician believed the patient may have sustained a right rotator cuff injury. The medical decision was straightforward in complexity.

a. 99255
b. 99283
c. 99253
d. 99221

70. An established patient is seen in a nursing facility by the physician because the patient, who is a diabetic, has developed a Stage II decubitus ulcer with cellulitis. The physician performs a detailed history and examination. The medical decision making complexity is moderate. The physician revises the patient's medical care plan.

a. 99310
b. 99309
c. 99315
d. 99218

71. The provider performed an internet assessment for ten minutes, visited three other patients for 5 minutes each, then came back and finished the session for another 20 minutes. The provider called the requesting physician and verbally reviewed the call. Code for this service.

a. 99446
b. 99447
c. 99448
d. This is not a reportable service.

72. A 60-year-old male presents for a complete physical. There are no new complaints since my previous examination on June 9 of last year. The patient spends 6 hours a week golfing and reports a brisk and active retirement. He does not smoke and has only an occasional glass of wine. He sleeps well but has been having nocturia times three. On physical examination, the patient is a well- developed, well-nourished male. The physician continues and provides a complete examination of the patient lasting 45 minutes.

a. 99396
b. 99386
c. 99403
d. 99450

Anesthesia

73. What modifier would be used to code the physical status for a patient who had a mild systemic disease?

a. P1
b. P2
c. P3
d. P5

74. The qualifying circumstances code indicates a 75-year-old male.

a. 99100
b. 99140
c. 99116
d. 99135

75. This type of sedation decreases the level of the patient's alertness but allows the patient to cooperate during the procedure.

a. Topical
b. Local
c. Regional
d. Conscious

76. What publication is the National Unit Values published?

a. BVR by AS
b. RVG by ASA
c. ASA by RVG
d. RVP by ASA

77. To calculate the unit value of services for two procedures performed on the same patient during the same operative session you would do the following to report anesthesia services.

a. Report only the units for the highest unit value procedure.
b. Report only the units for the lowest unit value procedure.
c. Subtract the procedure with the lowest unit value from the procedure with the highest unit value.
d. Add the units of the two procedures together.

78. Code anesthesia service provided for an anterior cervical discectomy with decompression of a single interspace of the spinal cord and nerve roots and including osteophytectomy

a. 00620
b. 00640
c. 00630
d. 00600

79. Per CPT guidelines, anesthesia time ends:

a. When the patient leaves the operating room
b. When the anesthesiologist is no longer in personal attendance on the patient.
c. When the patient has fulfilled post anesthesia care unit criteria for recovery
d. When the patient leaves the post anesthesia care unit.

80. A physical status anesthesia modifier of P4 means that a patient has:

a. Has a mild systemic disease
b. Has a severe systemic disease
c. Has a severe systemic disease that is a constant threat of life
d. Is moribund

81. Qualifying circumstances anesthesia codes are used:

a. In addition to the anesthesia.
b. To describe circumstances that impact the character of the anesthesia
c. To describe provision of anesthesia under particularly difficult circumstances.
d. All of the above

82. Anesthesia time starts when:

a. When the Anesthesiologist meets the family
b. When the Anesthesiologist begins to administer drugs
c. When the Anesthesiologist prepares the patient for induction - preoperative
d. When the Anesthesiologist comes to work

Radiology

83. A 60-year-old female comes to the clinic with shortness of breath. The Doctor orders a chest x-ray, frontal and lateral.

a. 71046 x 2, R06.2
b. 71047 x 2, R06.89
c. 71048, R06.09
d. 71046, R06.02

84. A patient presents for an MRI of the pelvis with contrast materials.

a. 72125
b. 72198
c. 72196
d. 72159

85. Code an endoscopic catheterization of the biliary ductal system for the professional radiology component only.

a. 74330-TC
b. 74330-26
c. 74328-26
d. 74300-26

86. Marcy is a 29-year-old pregnant female in for a follow-up ultrasound with image documentation of the uterus.

a. 76856
b. 74740
c. 76816
d. 74710

87. Code a complex brachytherapy isodose calculation for a patient with prostate cancer:

a. 77318, C61
b. 77317-22, C62.90
c. 77772, C52
d. 77300, C52

88. This patient received a prescription for a therapeutic radiology for a cancerous neoplasm of the adrenal gland. What code would you use for complex treatment planning?

a. 60520
b. 77307
c. 77401
d. 77263

89. Because of frequent headaches, this 50-year-old female's doctor ordered a CT scan of her head, without contrast materials.

a. 70450
b. 70460
c. 70470
d. 70496

Pathology and Laboratory

90. A patient presents to the laboratory in the clinic for the following tests: TSH, comprehensive metabolic panel, and an automated hemogram with manual differential WBC count (CBC). How would you code this lab?

a. 84445, 80051, 85025
b. 84443
c. 80050
d. 84443, 80053, 85027, 85007

91. An 81-year-old female patient presented to the laboratory for a lipid panel that includes measurement of total serum cholesterol, lipoprotein (direct measurement, HDL), and triglycerides.

a. 80061
b. 80061-52
c. 82465, 83718, 84478
d. 82465-52, 83718, 84478

92. Thomas has end stage renal failure and comes to the clinic lab today for his monthly urinalysis (qualitative, microscopic only).

a. 81015, N19
b. 81001, N17.9
c. 81015, N18.6
d. 81003, N18.6

93. This 34-year-old female had been suffering from chronic fatigue. Her physician has ordered a TSH test.

a. 80418, R53.81
b. 80438, R53.82
c. 84146, R53.81
d. 84443, R53.82

94. Surgical pathology, gross examination, or microscopic examination is most often required when a sample of an organ, tissue, or body fluid is taken from the body. What code(s) would you use to report biopsy of the colon, hematoma, pancreas, and a tumor of the testis?

a. 88307, 88304, 88309
b. 88305, 88304, 88307
c. 88305, 88302, 88307, 88309
d. 88305, 88304, 88307, 88309

95. This patient presents to the clinic lab for a prothrombin time measurement because of long-term use of Coumadin.

a. 85210, Z79.01
b. 85210, Z79.2
c. 85610, Z79.01
d. 85230, Z79.2

96. The 62-year-old female who suffers from treatment-resistant schizophrenia comes into the lab today to have a quantitative drug assay performed for the anti-psychotic medication clozapine, a regular white blood cell and absolute neutrophil count due to concern with agranulocytosis.

a. 80159
b. 80159, 85048
c. 80159, 85048, 85004
d. 80159, 85025

97. The 67-year-old female suffers from Chronic liver disease and needs a hepatic function panel performed every six months. Tests include total bilirubin (82274), direct bilirubin (82248), total protein (84155), alanin aminotransferases (ALT and SGPT) (84460), aspartate aminotransferases (AST and SGOT) (84450) and what other lab tests?

a. 82040, 84075
b. 80061, 83718
c. 82040, 82247
d. 84295, 84450

98. The patient presented to the laboratory at the clinic for the following blood tests ordered by her physician: albumin (serum), bilirubin (total), and Urea nitrogen (BUN) (quantitative)

a. 82044, 82248, 84520
b. 82040, 82252, 84525
c. 82040, 82247, 84520
d. 82044, 82247, 84540

99. This male is status post kidney transplant and comes into the clinic for a follow up creatinine clearance.

a. 82540, Z94.0
b. 82575, Z94.0
c. 82565, N19
d. 82570, N18.6

Medicine

100. An elderly man comes in for his flu (split virus, IM) and pneumonia (23-valent, IM) vaccines. Code only the immunization administration and diagnoses for the vaccines.

a. 90658, 90632, Z23, Z23
b. 90471, 90658, 90472, 90732, Z23, Z23
c. 90471 x 2, 90658, 90632, Z23
d. 90471, 90472, Z23, Z23

101. Code for a tetravalent, preservative free, flu vaccine for a three-year old girl, injected intramuscularly.

a. 90686
b. 90686, 90471
c. 90687, 90460
d. 90688, 90460

102. The established patient is seen for a comprehensive eye exam (not E & M), fundus photography and the application of corneal bandage lenses for Keratoconus. Code for this encounter.

a. 99215, 92250, 92082
b. 92004, 92250, 92072
c. 92014, 92250, 92071
d. 92014, 92250, 92072

103. The patient, a 55-year-old male. This was a follow up for POAG. The patient had IOP of 22 OD and 24 OS, The Optometrist added Timolol Maleate to the patient's Xalatan prescription. The OD performed a Comprehensive Eye Exam, which included ExtraOcular Motility (EOM) Confrontation Fields and a Dilated Fundus Exam, No ROS was taken. The provider performed a refraction exam and GDX of the retina of both eyes.

a. 99215, 92132
b. 92004, 92250, 92015
c. 92014, 92134, 92015
d. 92014, 92134

104. This 70-year-old male is taken to the emergency room with severe chest pain. The physician provided an expanded problem-focused history and examination. While the physician is examining the patient, his pressures drop and he goes into cardiac arrest. Cardiopulmonary resuscitation is given to the patient, and his pressure returns to normal; he is transferred to the intensive care unit in critical condition. Code the cardiopulmonary resuscitation and the diagnosis. The medical decision making was of low complexity.

a. 99282, 92950, I46.9
b. 99283, 92970, I46.9
c. 92950, I46.9
d. 92960, I46.9

105. A patient is taken to the OR for insertion of a Swan-Ganz catheter. The physician inserts the catheter for monitoring cardiac output measurements and blood gases.

a. 36013, 93503
b. 36013
c. 93451
d. 93503

106. Dr White orders a sleep study for Dan a 50-year-old male who has been diagnosed with obstructive sleep apnea. The sleep study will be done with C-PAP (continuous positive airway pressure).

a. 95806, R06.81
b. 95907, G47.30
c. 95807, G47.30
d. 95811, G47.33

107. Mary is a 50-year-old female with end-stage renal failure. She receives dialysis Tuesdays, Thursdays, and Saturdays each week. She sees the physician 4 times per month. Code a full month of dialysis for the month of December.

a. 90960 X4, N18.6
b. 90960, N18.6
c. 90960, N19
d. 90961, N19

108. OPERATIVE REPORT

PROCEDURE PERFORMED: Primary stenting of 70% proximal posterior descending artery stenosis.

INDICATIONS: Atherosclerotic heart disease

DESCRIPTION OF PROCEDURE: Stents inserted via percutaneous transcatheter placement. A 2.5 x 13 mm pixel stent was deployed.

COMPLICATIONS: None

RESULTS: Successful primary stenting of 70% proximal posterior descending artery stenosis with no residual stenosis at the end of the procedure.

a. 92920-RC, 92928, I25.10
b. 92920-RC, I25.9
c. 92928-RC, I25.10
d. 92933-RC, I25.10

109. Dr Green is a neuroradiologist who has taken Barry, a 42-year-old male, with a diagnosis of carotid stenosis, to the operating room to perform a thrombo-endarterectomy, unilateral. During the surgery, the patient is monitored by electroencephalogram (EEG). Code the monitoring only.

a. 95957
b. 95816
c. 95819
d. 95955

Section 3: Medical Concepts:

Medical Terminology

110. What part of the neuron receives signals?

a. Myelin sheath
b. Dendrites
c. Axon
d. Cell body

111. Which type of atelectasis is the most common?

a. Inflammation
b. Chronic
c. Compression
d. Absorption

112. What condition is symptomatic of an enlargement of the alveoli and loss of elasticity?

a. Asthma
b. Chronic bronchitis
c. Empyema
d. Emphysema

113. A malignant bone tumors called _____.

a. Rhabdomyosarcoma
b. Osteosarcoma
c. Multiple myeloma
d. Chondrosarcoma

114. Name a malignant cartilage-based tumor found in middle-aged and older people

a. Rhadbomyosarcoma
b. Osteosarcoma
c. Chondrosarcoma
d. Chondroblastoma

115. What is the condition called when one accumulates dust particles in the lungs?

a. Tuberculosis
b. Pneumoconiosis
c. Pleurisy
d. Chronic obstructive pulmonary disease

116. What is the condition called where pus is in the pleural space and is sometimes a complication of pneumonia?

a. Pneumothorax
b. Empyema
c. Cor pulmonale
d. Atelectasis

117. What is another name for a compound fracture?

a. Open fracture
b. Closed fracture
c. Complete fracture
d. Incomplete facture

118. Which of the following is NOT an ear bone?

a. Styloid
b. Incus
c. Stapes
d. Malleus

119. The term for a growth plate is?

a. Periosteum
b. Metaphysic
c. Epiphyseal
d. Endosteum

Anatomy

120. Which septum divides the upper two chambers of the heart?

a. Myocardium
b. Intraventricular
c. Tricuspid
d. Interatrial

121. What condition has predominant symptoms of rapid, involuntary eye movement?

a. Astigmatism
b. Nystagmus
c. Diplopia
d. Hyperopia

122. Bacterial cystitis is usually caused by?

a. Staphylococci
b. Proteus
c. Pseudomonas
d. E. Coli

123. Which below is located in a depression in the skull at the base of the brain:

a. Thymus
b. Pituitary
c. Pineal
d. Adrenal

ICD-10-CM

124. The patient, a four-year old child, complained of pain from inside her ear. The doctor found a retained glass fragment in the child's ear.

a. H92.09, H74.8x9, Z18.83
b. H92.09, H74.8x9, Z18.81
c. H92.09, H74.43, Z18.81
d. H92.09, H69.80, Z18.81

125. Acute Bacterial endocarditis due to AIDS.

a. B20, I33.0
b. B20, I39
c. B20, I33.9
d. A80.39, I39

126. Asymptomatic, non-sustained, ventricular tachycardia, there are no prolonged pauses, predominant rhythm is atrial fibrillation with well-controlled ventricular rate.

a. I48.92, I42.8
b. I48.91, I42.8
c. I49.01, I42.8
d. I42.8, I48.91

127. A 50-year-old female patient had two separate carbuncles removed from the left axilla. Pathology report indicated staphylococcal infection.

a. L02.432, B95.8
b. L02.92, B95.5
c. L02.92, B95.4
d. L02.432, B95.7

128. A 55-year-old female with spinal stenosis of the cervical disk C4-5 and C5-6 with inter-vertebral disk displacement had a cervical discectomy, corpectomy, allograft from C4 to C6 and placement of arthrodesis (a 34 mm plate from C4 to C6)

a. M50.90
b. M48.02, M50.221, M50.222
c. M48.02, M51.26
d. M50.90, M51.35

129. A 50-year-old male has staphylococcal septicemia with systemic inflammatory response syndrome and respiratory and hepatic failure

a. A41.2, J96.00, K72.00
b. A41.2, J96.00, R65.20
c. J96.00, K72.00, A40.8, R65.20
d. A41.2, R65.20, J96.00, K72.00

130. The patient, a 21-year old female, has acute laryngitis, chronic fatigue syndrome and presents for both the FLU and pneumococcal vaccine.

a. Z22.9, J04.0, R53.83
b. Z23, Z23, J37.0, R53.81
c. Z22.9, Z23, J37.1, R53.81
d. Z23, Z23, J04.0, R53.82

131. A 5-year-old patient is seen by a physician in an outpatient clinic for chronic lymphoid leukemia in remission and Shiga toxin-producing Escherichia coli:

a. C91.11, B96.21
b. C91.Z1, A04.4
c. C92.21, A41.51
d. C91.Z1, B96.20

132. Discharged with Pneumonia, klebsiella pneumoniae, COPD with emphysema, multifocal atrial tachycardia, middle dementia.

a. J15.0, J43.9, I49.8, F06.8
b. J15.20, J43.9, I49.8, F06.8
c. J18.9, J43.9, I49.8, F06.8
d. J18.9, J43.9, I49.8, F02.81

133. A patient with a history of myocardial infarction is admitted for cardiac catheterization. It is also noted the patient has unstable angina, hypertension, and diabetes with hypoglycemia.

a. I20.0, I10, E13.9, D10.9
b. I20.8, I10, E11.69, I25.2
c. I20.0, I10, E11.69, I25.2
d. I20.0, I10, I21.3, E11.69, I25.2

HCPCS

134. Level II HCPCS codes for drugs are administered:

a. Intravenously
b. Intramuscularly
c. Subcutaneously
d. All of the above

135. A male 62-year-old presents for a digital rectal exam and total prostate-specific antigen test (PSA), which code would is used?

a. G0102
b. G0103
c. G0102, G0106
d. G0102, G0103

136. A Medicare patient, 82-year-old female has an energy x-ray absorptiometry (SEXA) bone density study of two sites of the wrists.

a. G0141
b. G0143
c. G0130
d. G0129

137. A 63-year-old male, Medicare recipient receives 30 minutes of individual diabetes outpatient self-management training:

a. G0109
b. G0176
c. 99213
d. G0108

138. A Medicare recipient presents for an influenza and pneumococcal vaccination.

a. G0008
b. G0009
c. G0008, G0009
d. G0010, G0008

139. General guidelines for HCPCS Level II Coding include:

a. Code directly from the index
b. Search for main terms and any applicable sub-terms
c. Note the reference codes as given in the index
d. All of the above.

Coding Guidelines

140. A separate procedure is coded per CPT guidelines:

a. Is considered to be an integral part of a larger service
b. Is coded when it is performed as a part of another, larger procedure
c. Is never coded under any circumstances
d. Both A and B are correct

141. The symbol TRIANGLE before a code in the CPT manuals means?

a. The code is exempt from bundling requirements
b. The code has been revised in some way this year.
c. The code is exempt from unbundling requirements.
d. The code can be used as an add-on code, never reported alone or first.

142. Which is true of the CPT code(s):

a. They describe non-physician services
b. They are numeric
c. Only physicians can report them
d. All of the above are correct

143. CPT has been developed and maintained by _____.

a. AMA
b. CMS
c. The Cooperating Parties
d. WHO

144. This group performs the daily operations for CMS.

a. OIG
b. PRO
c. FI (and carriers)
d. WHO

145. When using the ICD-10-CM

a. Always use the index only when coding
b. Check the tabular before assigning a code
c. It is perfectly appropriate to memorize codes
d. B and C are correct

146. ICD-10-CM codes are composed of 3-7 alpha and numeric digit codes, when using them:

a. Code to the greatest detail
b. It is appropriate to code the 3 digit code when the category is further defined
c. Code to the 4th digit when you don't have the information in your notes
d. B and C are correct

147. When Acute and Chronic Conditions are noted:

a. Always code the Chronic Condition first
b. Always code the Acute Condition first
c. Code both and sequence the acute (sub-acute) code first
d. B and C are correct

148. Which is not true of Z-Codes

a. Must always be used at primary diagnosis
b. Are used for other reasons for the encounter
c. Describe signs & symptoms
d. Used to classify diseases and injuries

Billing

149. What tool is in place that manages multiple third-party payments to ensure that over-payment does not happen?

a. FUD
b. DME
c. COB
d. PRO

150. A PAR provider:

a. Signs an agreement with the Fiscal Intermediary
b. Submits charges directly to CMS
c. Receives 5% less than some other providers
d. Can bill the patient after payment from Medicare

CPC Mock Exam - Answers and Rationale

Section 1: Surgery and Modifiers:

10,000 series

1. a. S51.012A, L03.114, cellulitis secondary to superficial injury, always code the additional injury or ulcer code B95.5, always code bacterial agents after the disease manifestation. 99201 minimal E & M visit for a new patient. Injection, IM, 96372, J0561 X 12, always code the drug and administration of the drug times amount of drug used.

2. d. S81.012A, key word laceration, knee. S61.411A, key word: laceration; right hand. W01.110A, Y92.099, Code location and instrument, 12032, 12004-51 code location and size adding together the wounds in the same location regardless how many. Remember that simple closure and single layer are considered the same type of closure.

3. a. C44.329, key word: carcinoma, squamous cell. D17.22, Lipomas are benign and coded by site. 11641-RT, malignant lesion removals are coded separately by site. 11403-51-LT, 12031-51-LT skin lesion removal includes simple repair, code intermediate or layered closures. Both codes are required. See surgery guidelines.

4. d. 15100-LT, 15002-51-LT. code both the wound preparation and then any intermediate graft.

5. c. C44.319, Carcinoma, basal cell of skin of other parts of face. 15120, key word split-thickness. 11646 excision of a malignant lesion.

6. c. T83.511A, N39.0, B96.20, always code reason for the encounter and any manifestations. Y84.6, code the cause 51702 Insertion of temporary indwelling catheter simple.

7. a. A82.9, S61.429A, W55.51XA, Y07.12, T76.92XA, code manifestation and cause codes. 99291, key word critical care for 60 minutes. 92950, Key word; CPR. Be sure to read the guidelines and highlight what is included in critical care services.

8. d 12051 Repair intermediate, wound face.

9. c. 15271-RT; 15271-LT, 15272-LT Application of skin substitute graft to trunk, arms, legs, total wound surface area up to 100 sq cm; first 25 sq cm or less wound surface area (2012) 15272 is the ADD-ON code for the left leg. Often with skin grafts, specific types and brands are identified and have to be cross-linked to the CPT definition. Biobrane: For use in clean and non-infected, superficial partial-thickness burns with minimal involvement of the dermis.

10. d. 10005, 10006: These codes were added in 2019. Key term is "fine needle aspiration;", Use code 1005 for first biopsy and 1006 for second breast. No modifier is needed.

20000 Series

11. d. 28406-LT key words, manipulated, percutaneous fixation, left heel.

12. a. 27200, open manipulation was never mentioned. The default is to code as closed.

13. d. 27252-LT key words: under anesthesia and pressure.

14. d. 27538-LT key words: fracture, tibial, tuberosity.

15. a. 28545-LT key words: under general anesthesia, dislocation, left tarsal.

16. c. 20661 application of halo, including removal: cranial.

17. b. 20520-LT key words: lodged in muscle, without complication.

18. b. 23030-RT key words: deep, hematoma.

19. d. 22633 Arthrodesis, combined posterior or posterolateral technique with posterior interbody technique including laminectomy and/or discectomy sufficient to prepare interspace (other than for decompression), single interspace and segment; lumbar 22634 is the ADD-ON code for each additional interspace and segment. (Note: 22634 states AMA guidelines "Use 22634 in conjunction with 22633")

20. b. 29425-RT, application of walking cast; S93.402A, sprain left lower leg; W06.xxxA fall from bed, code location as Bedroom of single-family (private) house: Y92.013.

21. a. 12002-RT simple wound of the extremity. Select for size, location and type. This might be considered a trick question because it is in the 20000 section but that will happen on an actual test.

22. b. 12032 key words: right arm and deep. size of wound.

23. b. 12041-RT intermediate repair; 12002-RT simple repair, Report modifier 51 for second procedure.

30000 Series

24. d. 33536, 4 or more coronary arterial grafts, 33522, an add-on code primary procedure first (AMA "Use in conjunction with 33533-33536), I25.10, native vessels were specified.

25. b. 36620, separate procedure code.

26. c. 38115, repair ruptured spleen D73.5, Infarction of spleen includes splenic rupture non-traumatic. There is no mention that it is laparoscopic.

27. d. 36571, 77001, Fluoroscopic guidance is not included in service.

28. d. 33366-LT is the correct code. Transcatheter aortic valve replacement (TAVR/TAVI) with prosthetic valve; transapical exposure (eg, left thoracotomy).

29. a. One. Per the CPT Guidelines for this section use a single interventional code, 37230, for the femoral/popliteal territory and do not use Add-On codes. Read and highlight all guidelines notes.

30. a. 30520, 30140-51, Septoplasty, per notes below the code, does not include turbinate resection; J34.2, deviated septum.

31. a. 31255, 31267-51, ethmoidectomy excludes antrostomy must report both codes; J32.9, chronic sinusitis unspecified. See notes below the code. (AMA Guidelines: Do not report 31256, 31267 in conjunction with 31295 when performed on the same sinus)

40000 Series

32. a. 47562, Laparoscopy, surgical; cholecystectomy

33. c. 44960 key words, appendix, ruptured, generalized peritonitis.

34. c. 43262, endoscopic retrograde cholangiopancrateography with sphincterotomy/papillotomy. (AMA Guidelines: 43262 may be reported when sphincterotomy is performed in addition to 43261, 43263, 43264, 43265, 43275, 43278. Do not report 43262 in conjunction with 43274 for stent placement or with 43276 for stent replacement [exchange] in the same location. Do not report 43262 in conjunction with 43260, 43277)

35. d. Query the physician as to the method used is the best answer.

36. b. 42420-80, total removal with perseveration of the facial nerve; use modifier 80 to show that you are coding for the assistant. D49.89, Neoplasm of unspecified nature of other specified sites.

37. a. 42825, tonsillectomy; J35.01, Chronic tonsillitis

38. a. 45303, proctosigmoidoscopy with dilation

39. d. 45338, code to the farthest placement of the scope and include removal of neoplasm if present; D12.5 benign neoplasm of the sigmoid colon

40. a. 46250, complete removal of hemorrhoids; K64.4, external removal without mention of complication.

50000 Series

41. a. 50200-50, key words percutaneous needle.

42. b. 52204, cystourethroscopy with biopsy

43. d. 52450, 52000-59, must use modifier 59 and documentation must support the separate and distinct nature of both codes, to support the cystoscopy (separate procedure) N32.0 Bladder obstruction.

44. a. 54300 for straightening of chordee (e.g., hypospadias).

45. d. 54150-52, See notes below the code; add MODIFIER-52 when performed without dorsal penile or ring block

46. c. 55250, code is listed as unilateral and bilateral

47. d. 56420, Incision and drainage of Bartholin's gland abscess.

48. a. 57455, Colposcopy of the cervix including upper/adjacent vagina; with biopsy(s) of the cervix

49. a. 59121, no mention of salpingectomy and/or oophorectomy.

50. d. 59515, Cesarean delivery only; including postpartum care

51. b. 58120, excludes postpartum hemorrhage

52. c. 55100, key word: drain.

60000 Series

53. a. 60254, key word: total; C73, Malignant neoplasm of thyroid gland.

54. c. 61150, keyword: drain.

55. a. 61710, keywords: balloon catheter.

56. d. 67938, removal of embedded foreign body, eyelid.

57. c. 69436-50, key word: insertion of ventilating tubes, (For bilateral procedure, report 69436 with MODIFIER 50); H66.93, otitis media, unspecified, bilateral.

58. b. 69424-50, report bilateral procedure (MODIFIER-50) when physician performs procedure on both sides at the same operative session.

59. d. 69603, keywords radical mastoidectomy. NOT modified or complete.

60. d. 67810-E1 always code location with modifier. However, in the real world most carriers only accept RT and LT for epilation, not the E1-E4 modifiers.

61. b. 67311, keyword: lateral.

62. c. 67961, keyword: one-forth.

Section 2: E/M; Radiology, Path & Lab, Medicine

Evaluation and Management

63. c. 99203, Key words: 90-year old means do not report an E & M consultation code to Medicare, report as a new patient. Also, the physician was charged with diagnosing the patient. Do not bill a consult visit when the patient asks for the second opinion. Detailed Hx and Exam and Medical Decision Making of low complexity = 99203.

64. a. 99223, Key words attending physician, high complexity, comprehensive history

65. c. 99255, Key words; inpatient, comprehensive history, Comprehensive physical examination.

66. b. 99282; Key word; expanded problem focused, low complexity medical decision making and emergency department.

67. b. 99325, Key words: new patient, custodial care center, expanded problem focused, and Medical Decision Making, low.

68. b. 99219, admitted for observation; use the facility observation visit (99217-99220); comprehensive history, Medical Decision Making, Moderate Complexity. E&M Code 99225 are "Out of Order" Codes since the 99221 - 99223 were already taken.

69. d. 99221, Key words: admitted to hospital after car accident, lets you know that it is an initial visit. Detailed history and straightforward medical decision making.

70. b. 99309, Key words: established, nursing facility, detailed history and exam, Medical Decision Making is moderate in complexity.

71. d. The break in time is meant as a distraction. They key to the answer is that there is no mention of a written report, which is required for all the new 2014 interprofessional telephone/Internet assessment E & M codes. Therefore, this is not a reportable service. If the written report was performed it would have been a 99448 code, adding both times.

72. a. 99396, periodic comprehensive preventive medicine reevaluation and management including age and gender appropriate history, examination (age 40-64). Also called a Annual Wellness Exam or Routine Medical Exam.

Anesthesia

73. b. P2, a patient with mild systemic disease.

74. a. 99100, patient of extreme age and younger than 1 year and older than 70.

75. d. Conscious Sedation means the patient can respond to commands. Combinations of pharmacological agents administered by one or more routes to produce a minimally depressed level of consciousness and satisfactory analgesia while retaining the ability to independently and continuously maintain an airway and respond to physical stimulation and verbal commands. Examples of regional blocks include spinals, epidurals or peripheral nerve blocks.

76. b. RVG (Relative Value Guide) by ASA (American Society of Anesthesiologists).

77. a. Report only the units for the highest unit value procedure.

78. d. 00600, Anesthesia for procedures on cervical spine and cord; not otherwise specified.

79. b. When the anesthesiologist is no longer in personal attendance on the patient.

80. c. Has a severe systemic disease that is a constant threat of life.

81. d. Always use qualifying circumstance modifiers in addition to the anesthesia service, when circumstances impact the character of the anesthesia, or to describe provisions that that render anesthesia under particularly difficult circumstances.

82. c. When the Anesthesiologist prepares the patient for induction - preoperative.

Radiology

83. d. 71046, radiologic examination, chest, 2 views, frontal and lateral. R06.02, shortness of breath.

84. c. 72196, Magnetic resonance imaging, pelvis; with contract materials(s).

85. c. 74328-26, interpretation of, Endoscopic catheterization of the biliary ductal system, radiological supervision and interpretation.

86. c. 76816, Ultrasound, pregnant uterus, real time with image documentation, follow-up.

87. a. 77318, Brachytherapy isodose plan complex, C61, Malignant neoplasm of the prostate.

88. d. 77263, keyword(s); therapeutic radiology treatment planning, complex.

89. a. 70450, Computed tomography, head or brain; without contrast material.

Path and Lab

90. c. 80050, general health panel, includes DBD, comprehensive metabolic profile, CBC automated and appropriate manual differential WBC count TSH.

91. a. 80061, lipid panel includes cholesterol, serum, total lipoprotein, direct measurement, high density cholesterol.

92. c. 81015, Urinalysis, microscopic only, N18.6, end stage renal disease.

93. d. 84443, Thyroid Stimulating Hormone (TSH), R53.82, chronic fatigue syndrome.

94. d. 88305, 88304, 88307, 88309, surgical pathology code location from which biopsy was taken.

95. c. 85610, Prothrombin time Z79.01 encounter for long term (current) use of anticoagulants.

96. b. 80159: [2014 code] Clozapine; therapeutic drug assay for Clozapine. (This is quantitative; for nonquantitative testing see drug testing 80100-80104). In CPT, 85048 is listed as: Blood count; leukocyte (WBC), automated. Unless the coder works in a lab, this question can be very difficult as the information necessary to code it accurately is not in the CPT manual; additional information is needed. Neutrophil granulocytes are the most abundant type of white blood cells in humans and form an essential part of the immune system. Diagnostic labs also list code 85048 as Absolute Neutrophil Count (ANC), Blood. Both Quest diagnostics and Geisinger medical laboratories consider the one code (85048) sufficient to report both the White Blood Cell (WBC) and the absolute neutrophil cell (ANC) count. The CBC, 85025, and adding code 85004 would be unnecessary.

97. a. 82040, Albumin: serum, plasma or whole blood. 84075, phosphatase, alkaline.

98. c. 82040, Albumin: serum, plasma or whole blood, 82247, Bilirubin, total, 84520, Urea nitrogen (BUN): quantitative.

99. b. 82575, Creatinine; clearance, Z94.0, kidney replaced by transplant.

Medicine

100. d. 90471, 1st administration. 90472, 2nd administration, Z23, need for influenza vaccine, Z23, need for pneumococcal vaccine.

101. b. 90686: Influenza virus vaccine, quadrivalent, split virus, preservative free, when administered to individuals 3 years of age and older, for intramuscular use. Quadrivalent (aka tetravalent) means the vaccine is a mixture of four flu-types. A "split virus" is chemically disrupted using a non-ionic surfactant, which is further purified. Bivalent is two and trivalent is three. Report the vaccine admin codes 90471-74 in addition to codes 90476-90749.

102. d 92014 comprehensive eye exam. 99250 Fundus photography. Note: for keratoconus. 92072 Fitting of contact lens for management of keratoconus, initial fitting.

103. c. Key Hints here: 55-year old is not a Medicare patient, POAG is Primary Angle Glaucoma, IOP is IntraOcular Pressure The Comprehensive Eye exam is a 92014 code and not an E & M code. Clues are the two included tests (EOM and CF) and that no ROS was done (not need for 92xxx codes) GDX HRT and OCT are all diagnostic tests coded as Scanning Computerized Ophthalmic Diagnostic Imaging (SCODI) 9213x, 92134 is the correct code. Code 92015 for the refraction services. Determination of refractive state.

104. c. 92950, Cardiopulmonary resuscitation (eg, in cardiac arrest) I46.9, cardiac arrest, cause unspecified.

105. d. 93503, insertion and placement of flow directed catheter (eg. Swan-Ganz) for monitoring purposes.

106. d. 95811, polysomnography; sleep staging with 4 or more additional parameters of sleep, with initiation of continuous positive airway pressure (C-PAP) therapy or bi-level ventilation attended by a technologist, G47.33, obstructive sleep apnea (adult) (pediatric).

107. b. 90960, ESRD, for patients 20 years of age or older, N18.6, End stage renal failure, Chronic Kidney Disease.

108. c. 92928-RC, Modifier for right coronary artery, Transcatherter placement of an intracoronary stent(s). I25.10, Coronary atherosclerosis.

109. d. 95955, EEG during nonintracranial surgery (eg. Carotid surgery)

Section 3: Medical Concepts:

Medical Terminology

110. b. Dendrites are the afferent branches of the soma that receives signals.

111. b. Chronic. Atelectasis is the collapse of part or [much less commonly] all of a lung. A chronic form, designated middle lobe syndrome, results from compression of the middle lobe bronchus by surrounding lymph nodes.

112. d. Emphysema, a chronic pulmonary disease.

113. b. Osteosarcoma, a malignant sarcoma of the bone.

114. c. Chondrosarcoma a malignant tumor of the cartilage.

115. b. Pneumoconiosis; a condition of the respiratory tract due to inhalation of dust particles.

116. b. Empyema; a collection of pus in a body cavity (especially in the lung cavity).

117. a. Open, fracture of bone where broken end of bone had penetrated the skin.

118. a. Styloid.

119. c. Epiphyseal, means growth.

Anatomy

120. d. Interatrial, located between the atrial of the heart.

121. b. Nystagmus, movement may be in any direction. Etiology; may be congenital and in apparent to the patient; seen in bilateral amblyopia.

122. d. E. Coli; Escherichia coli.

123. b. Pituitary, also called the master gland.

ICD-10

124. b. H92.09: otogenic pain - of or originating within the ear, especially from inflammation of the ear. For H74.8x9 see Notes. Z18.81, retained glass fragments.

125. a. B20, HIV. I33.0 Acute and subacute infective endocarditis (use additional code to identify organism)

126. b. I48.91; unspecified atrial fibrillation, always code the reason for the encounter first. I42.8, other primary cardiomyopathies.

127. a. L02.432, B95.8; when coding L02 also identify the infective organism such as staphylococcus.

128. b. M48.02, M50.221, M50.222 mid-cervical region; keyword: displacement.

129. d. A41.2, R65.20, J96.00, K72.00; always code organism first then SIRS, followed by other manifestations.

130. d. Z23 is correct for influenza (flu), Z23 is the pneumococcal vaccine. R53.82 is chronic fatigue. J04.0 is acute laryngitis without mention of obstruction.

131. a. C91.11; key; in remission, B96.21: Shiga Toxin-producing Escherichia Coli [E coli] (STEC)

132. a. J15.0, Pneumonia due to Klebsiella pneumoniae ; J43.9, other emphysema; I49.8, other specified cardiac dysrhythmia; F06.8. Other specified mental disorders due to known physiological condition.

133. d. I20.0, Unstable angina; I10, Essential (primary) hypertension; I21.3, Acute myocardial infarction, episode of care unspecified; E11.69, Type 2 diabetes mellitus with other specified complication, code also the manifestation; I25.2, old myocardial infarction.

HCPCS

134. d. All of the Above. All codes are drug codes.

135. d. G0102, G0103; code digital rectal examination and prostate-specific antigen test. These are Medicare HCPC codes. Individual carriers may vary but coding exams are not reimbursement motivated.

136. c. G0130, code is a Medicare code. SEXA (Single energy x-ray absorptiometry bone density study).

137. d. G0108, code encounter for diabetes training.

138. c. G0008, G0009, code for each vaccination using Medicare payable codes.

139. b. Search for main terms and any applicable sub-terms.

Coding Guidlines

140. a. Is considered to be an integral part of a larger service; these codes can stand alone and can only be coded with a larger procedure when done at another location deeming it completely separate and using a modifier 59 to get paid for it.

141. b. The code description has been revised.

142. a. They describe both physician and non-physician services. Category II and III CPT Codes are alphanumeric with a T or F at the end.

143. a. AMA.

144. c. FI (and carriers); Fiscal Intermediary.

145. b. ALWAYS Check the tabular before assigning a code.

146. a. Code to the greatest detail.

147. c. Code both and sequence the acute (sub-acute) code first.

148. a. Must always be used as primary diagnosis.

Billing

149. c. COB; Coordination of Benefits.

150. a. Signs an agreement with FI.

Secrets To Reducing Exam Stress

What is Stress

Stress is a normal physical response to events that make you feel threatened or upset your balance in some way, such as situations beyond your control.

The body reacts to these situations with physical, mental, and emotional responses that all merge to create what is known as stress.

When you sense danger or events beyond your control the body's defense mechanisms kick into high gear causing a built in chain reaction of events to occur. This is natural for all of us.

Remember the first time someone reprimanded you for something you had done wrong? Not necessarily a parent or relative, but someone in school or at your place of employment where you felt threatened and began feeling stressed and nervous? That was a natural reaction to a set of circumstances that caused you to feel the effects of stress.

This can be a good thing during an emergency or other event but can also be a bad thing when you are trying to concentrate or think clearly for long periods of time, such as during an exam.

What Causes Stress and Anxiety

Stress is caused by fear, plain and simple. The fear of the unknown. The fear of failing. The fear of being unprepared. The fear of loss. The fear of an uncontrollable situation.

Anything beyond our control can cause fear or a sense of danger and this causes the body to release stress hormones, thus increasing your stress and anxiety level.

There are other factors that cause stress too including family, income, job, friends, life situations and others but the main focus of this book is stress directly attributed to exam preparation and taking an exam.

Once you learn how to reduce and manage stress for an exam you can certainly expand its uses to other areas of your life as well. As a matter of fact, I highly recommend that you do. The facts are clear, the less stress you have in your life the longer you will live and the better quality of life you will have.

What Are The Side Effects Of Stress

When stress is not controlled it can cause a significant amount of problems for people taking an exam. You have likely already experienced some of the side effects of stress including:

- Memory Problems

- Lack of Concentration

- Poor Judgement

- Negative Thoughts

- Headaches

- High Blood Pressure

- Upset Stomach

Each of these side effects can affect your exam preparation efforts and performance. As a matter of fact, in some extreme cases it can cause people to "lock up" and have difficulty even taking an exam. These cases are rare but they do exist. If you suffer from this type of reaction you know all too well how difficult it is to perform under these conditions, let alone excel or perform well enough to earn a passing grade.

So how can you control or minimize the effects of stress and even make it work for you?

Learn to Relax

Setting your mind at ease and learning how to relax can reduce stress dramatically. This is much easier said than done, however, there are different techniques to help you relax and each have there own set of benefits.

There are many different ways to relax your mind and body. Some are more difficult than others. Let's begin with an easy way to reduce even the most sever cases of stress.

Slow Breathing

When you begin to feel the effects of stress your breathing accelerates and your heart rate quickens. This is caused by adrenaline being pumped into your system from the body's reaction to a circumstance or situation.

The first thing you have to do is recognize that you are experiencing stress. After you have done that, the easiest and fastest way to reduce your stress level is to slow your breathing.

If you have ever watched a sporting event you have probably seen top athletes using this method to slow their heart rate, reduce adrenaline flow, relax their muscles, and clear their minds.

This helps them think more clearly, react more rapidly, and perform at a higher level. This is exactly what you want to do.

Top athletes do this when adrenaline is not a good thing and can effect performance.

A good example of this is golf. A golfer relies heavily on muscle memory to produce accurate and consistent golf shots. When adrenaline is introduced into their system, say during the final round of a tournament, it can cause a variation in the distance they hit the ball.

This can make them inconsistent at the very time when they need to be the most consistent.

And at the same time... with the stress level now amped up it can cause a player who normally makes sound decisions to now make questionable ones. This is strikingly similar to an exam situation.

Give this method a try. Take a deep breath and exhale slowly. Repeat this several times until your muscles are totally relaxed and your heart rate slows.

Use this method before studying and prior to and during the exam itself! It will help you think more clearly and be able to recall learned information more rapidly. This technique should be the first thing you do when you start to feel anxious or stressed.

> **"SOMETIMES WHEN PEOPLE ARE UNDER STRESS THEY HATE TO THINK, AND IT'S THE TIME THEY MOST NEED TO THINK."**
>
> **PRESIDENT BILL CLINTON**

Meditation

Please don't be intimidated by the word "meditation". It is not something to fear, rather something to embrace once you know a little more about it.

Meditation can give your mind a chance to take a much needed break, to "shut down", relax and recharge.

The biggest misconception about meditation is that it is something complex. It isn't. It is simply the process of relaxing your mind and body to give it a much needed break. This is exactly what you need to relieve stress.

Time to Meditate

Meditation does not take that long to do and it can be immensely valuable for your mind, body, and spirit. Scheduling a time to meditate is the best way to make sure it happens on a regular basis.

Set aside ten minutes prior to your scheduled study time each day to meditate. This will get you into the routine of doing it. Also schedule ten to twenty minutes prior to taking an exam to meditate when possible. It will help you relax and open your mind for better memory retention during study time and better information recall during exam time.

Meditation Exercises

Follow these simple steps to enjoy a deeper sense of relaxation.

- Sit in a relaxed position.
- Close your eyes.
- Rest your hands, palms up, on your lap.
- Breathe slowly and slightly deeper than normal.

- Concentrate on your breath coming in and going out.
- Quiet your mind. If you are thinking of something try to release the thought and concentrate on breathing again.
- As you become relaxed repeat a calming word or phrase such as "I feel calm" or "I can achieve", or even "I am the best".
- After ten minutes open your eyes slowly.

This should thoroughly relax you and give you positive thoughts and energy. Now your mind is free to accept new information when studying and ready to recall learned information more rapidly and accurately when taking an exam.

Meditation is nothing more than focused relaxation for the mind and body. Look at it this way. You rest your body six to eight hours per night. Sometimes your mind is resting but not always. So your mind doesn't get as much rest as your body does, just as everything else, it needs rest to be able to perform at a high level.

This is good for daily use, but *ultra* effective prior to exam preparation and before an actual exam.

Set Up A Routine

One of the most important actions you can take to reduce stress and anxiety is set up a study routine.

By setting up a regular study routine you remove the stress of trying to find time everyday to study. Schedule the time in advance. Commit to it and stick to it.

You know what time you have to go to work everyday... right? Why not know what time you are going to study everyday? All good habits are scheduled and repeated. Study time should be no different.

Scheduling

The best time to lay out a schedule is about a month to forty five days prior to an exam when possible. All exams are different but mapping out a consistent plan is essential. This is your way to say "this is important to me".

This will give you enough time to review all the material in a timely manner without cramming it all in at the last minute. This alone will reduce your stress level significantly as well as boost your confidence.

How Often Should You Study

A good study routine should consist of regularly scheduled short periods of uninterrupted and focused study time every day. This will give you time to absorb the information when you are alert and can concentrate fully.

Your study time should _not_ consist of hours upon hours of study time in one day and then no study time for several days. This will wear you down and reduce your ability to retain and recall information.

The last minute "all nighter" is the worst thing you can do! This time should only be for a last minute review of the most difficult material.

Plodding through hundreds of pages of information the night before an exam will only deprive you of sleep you desperately need and dilute any information you have already committed to memory.

You might occasionally "luck out" on an exam this way but keep in mind how much better you could have done had you prepared the right way.

How Long Should You Study

The ideal daily study time is an hour to two hours per day maximum! This will ultimately depend on your work, home, family, or school schedule of course but try to arrange something as close to this as possible.

If you schedule four to five hours or more in one day you are most likely defeating the purpose and wasting your time as your retention will start to decrease in hours three and beyond.

This is specially true if you have other commitments that require your time. Scheduling three or more hours of study time per day can actually add MORE stress to your life and reduce your sleeping time.

Either way this is exactly what you want to avoid at all costs! And I do mean ALL COSTS!

Scheduling time each day will keep you mentally fresh and absorbing good information PLUS it will give you the proper time for other commitments too! The outcome... reduce stressed.

Study With A Buddy

Whenever possible try to study with a buddy. Each person brings a different perspective to the learning process. This is a good way to retain new information because you are more focused on the task at hand when you are with someone else.

Plus, when you commit to study with a buddy the chances are you will actually follow through with your scheduled study time. No one likes to break a promise or commitment.

Commitment

Committing to study with a buddy is kind of like working out. It is hard to get motivated and push yourself to workout daily by yourself. That is just a fact. Only the most disciplined people can do this on their own and even some times they find it a challenge.

When you commit to meet a friend to workout it is much easier to keep your routine and commitment. Even though you may not want to workout that day, you recall the commitment you made to your friend and off you go to follow up on your commitment.

That commitment actually carries a lot of psychological weight with it. That is why people follow through with commitments made to others or in public and why it is important for you to commit to study with a buddy.

Plus the company never hurts either. Chances are you will both motivate each other to do more than you would have done alone.

The more you feel that you are not "in this alone" the more relaxed and confident you will be and the more you will get done.

Note: IMPORTANT**** *Study with a positive minded person. Don't get stuck listening to negative people and their excuses why they can't do this or that. These people are always looking to drag other people "down to their level" and are always reluctant to change to better themselves.*

If you arrange to study with a buddy and the person starts making negative comments... get out now! Don't waist your time trying to bring them up or convert them to your way of thinking.... it won't work! Stay positive and spend your time studying... not counseling. Leave that to the professionals.

Develop Your Concentration

Concentration is described as "intense mental application; complete attention".

It is your minds ability to focus on the task at hand and block out all other influences and distractions. To concentrate on one thing and one thing exclusively... the exam.

Information Retention

Your ability to concentrate is vital to your exam success. The more you concentrate on the subject materials the better you will retain and recall the information when the time comes to perform.

When you concentrate solely on the material it allows you less time to worry about other "stressors" or to give time for negative thoughts to enter in. And negative thoughts will try to work their way in. Self doubt is something that can be destructive so don't give your mind an opportunity to entertain negative thoughts.

For you to perform your best, all attention must be on the study material and the exam. This deep level of concentration will help you maximize your study time. In most cases, the better you can concentrate during your study time the less study time you will actually have to schedule. The saying "quality over quantity" applies to exam preparation too!

I mean... really, who wants to study for 5 hours at one sitting when you can study for 2 hours, with a high level of concentration and focus, and get the same results. No one. **Study Smarter, Not Longer!**

Benefits

Training your mind to concentrate on the task at hand will keep positive thoughts flowing and block out negative thoughts. Think of your mind as a bowl. You can only put so much in a bowl. So the more positive thoughts you put into the bowl the less room there is for negative ones.

Some of the benefits of increasing your level of concentration included:

- Peace of mind

- Self confidence

- Inner strength

- Ability to focus your mind

- Increased memory

- Ability to study and comprehend more quickly

- Less study time

Exercises

Here are some exercises to help you develop your concentration.

1) Select one thought and concentrate on it for ten minutes. This will be difficult at first but the more you do it the easier it will be to block out all other thoughts and concentrate on the one thought you have chosen.

2) Count the words in a paragraph. Count them again to ensure accuracy. Once you have completed this, count several paragraphs and then an entire page.

3) Take an object such as a spoon, fork, or anything out of a drawer. Try to concentrate on the object without mentally describing the object in words. Just focus on the object from all directions.

4) Draw a circle and color it in with any color. Now focus on the object and try not to think of any words, just focus on the object for several minutes.

5) Lie down and relax all your muscles. Once you are completely relaxed concentrated on your heartbeat and imagine your blood flowing throughout your body. After several minutes you should be able to feel the blood moving through your veins.

6) Watch the second hand on a clock. Focus just on the second hand and nothing else. Do this for two to three minutes and fight off the urge to let any other thoughts interfere with your concentration.

7) Close your eyes and visualize the number one. Say the number "one" in your head once you visualize it clearly. Now let it go and focus on the number two and repeat the process up to ten.

8) Take a coin out of your pocket. Relax every muscle in your body and concentrate on the coin and only the coin. View everything about it, its

shape, color, material makeup nicks, words. Now close your eyes and visualize the coin in full detail. If you can not visualize the coin in full detail open your eyes and try again.

9) Sit in a chair and relax. Focus on a spot on the wall and release all other thoughts from your mind. Now while looking at the spot on the wall focus on your breathing. Breath in slowly and then exhale slowly. Do this for several minutes.

10) Read an article in the newspaper. Capture the essentials of the article. Now describe the article in as few words as possible to a friend or just aloud to yourself.

Learning to concentrate fully on the task at hand is difficult but the benefits are enormous. It is easy to let your mind wander off and loose your train of thought during an exam.

The better your concentration is during your exam preparation the better your exam scores will be. It is as simple as that.

Concentration is critical, specially towards the end of the exam when it is easy to get distracted and lose focus as you start to get tired.

This is when this training will pay off. You will remain focused and keep your concentration though the entire exam.

Note: IMPORTANT** *These exercises are not for everyone, however, they are a valuable tool when learning to increase your concentration and mental focus.*

Try to do the exercises every other day. You will notice an increase in your information retention and recall. Plus this will help you study more efficiently and effectively!

Power of Positive Thinking

Positive thinking can reduce stress, improve your overall health, and make you much more interesting and fun to be around.

Although it is unclear exactly why positive thinkers experience health benefits, one of the theories is it helps them deal with stressful situations better. They are thinking of the best outcome, not the worst outcome, and this creates less stress and anxiety. This is better for the mind and the body.

I'll never forget an acquaintance of mine way back in the mid 80's who would shoot down new ideas like clay pigeons. Whenever a new idea would come up he would spend three times the intellectual effort to shoot it down than to consider if it would ever work. In his eyes "it would never work" no matter what it was.

Does that guy sound familiar to you? My guess is he probably does. You might have one or several people like this in your life right now. The best thing you can do is run... run... run.

I have nothing against shooting holes in a new idea to see if it stands the test of scrutiny, but just to dismiss a new idea because it represents change is unhealthy.

Negative people will try with all their might to bring you down. To make you surrender your positive "can do" attitude and keep them company in their pool of negativity. Don't let them!

Glass Half Full or Empty

Are you a "glass half full" or "glass half empty" type of person? Answering this question is a good way to find out if you are an optimist or a pessimist.

If you always see the good side of things (glass half full) then you are an optimist. If not, then you are a pessimist.

Optimists (or positive people) always consider the "what if it could work" side of things. They are happy and easy with a smile. They give as much positive energy as they get from others and are usually interesting and fun to be around.

An optimist is more likely to be successful too. They "will their self to victory". They tell THEMSELVES they can do something and this starts the ball of positivity and success rolling. Just as a snowball rolling down a mountain starts small, once it gains momentum there is little way to stop it.

Self Talk

Why is self talk important? Well, the mind is always thinking and creating "self-talk". Self-talk is the endless stream of thoughts that run through your head.

Self-talk is based on information, reason, logic, and prior experience. Self-talk also comes from misconceptions created because of misinformation or lack of information. This can be negative or positive, depending on your outlook.

For example, if someone asked you to jump over a hurdle and you've never jumped over a hurdle before, your mind would tell you either "you can do this" or "no way you can do this". This is commonly referred to as self-talk.

> "PROGRAM THE VOICE INSIDE YOUR HEAD. IT WILL LISTEN, YOU OWN IT."

Programing your self talk will help you control the way you look at things and the attitude you have towards them. Self-talk is enormously powerful and you want to have it on your side.

A good example of the power of self-talk became apparent to me while working out several years ago and its power and control made a lasting impression on me.

In 1998 I started to lap swim at the local YMCA. I started to lap swim for several reasons. First, to lose weight that had accumulated over years of sitting behind a desk and remaining inactive. And second, to relieve some of the stress that comes with an upper level management job that I had been promoted to several years before.

The process of building up to a meaningful workout was slow at first, only a swimming a few laps per session. But over time I had built up to swimming 27 laps (which equalled 3/4 of a mile) per session.

I stayed at that level for many years, mainly because I could get my workout in over an hour long lunch break. But a funny thing happened several years ago when I finally went to work for myself. And it was all brought to light while talking to fellow lap swimmer at the local YMCA.

Through conversation she asked "how far do you swim each day". I said "3/4 of a mile". She asked, "why don't you just swim a mile"? "I don't know" I replied. "I have been doing this for years and never gave it much thought".

The next time in the pool I tried to swim a mile (36 laps) and around lap number twenty my mind began telling me I was tired and it was almost time to quit.

And sure enough, at lap twenty seven I was in no position to go any further. I was done. My mind had convinced my body that 3/4 of a mile was enough for today.

It was hard to believe that my body just started to feel exhausted around the 3/4 mile mark, knowing full well I could swim more laps. So the next day I decided to control my self-talk and tell myself "I am going to swim thirty six laps today" and "I could do anything I put my mind to". I was literally trying to trick myself into thinking I could swim a full mile.

Swimming a full mile was not a problem that day because my mind was reinforcing the belief that I could swim a mile. By controlling my self-talk and keeping the self-talk positive instead of negative I was able to control the outcome and achieve more than what my mind had previously programed me to accept as my unconscious limit.

I have also used this technique to swim two miles in one session and lose over 60 pounds. Controlling your self-talk is powerful, and it works.

Unconscious Limits

Your mind sets unconscious limits for everything that you do based on previous experience and other inputs of information such as things you read or discuss with others. Your mind processes all this information to set predetermined limits for you.

This was exceptionally powerful when world class runners were trying to break the four minute mile mark. It was generally thought that no one could ever run a mile under four minutes.

And for years no one could surpass that mark until May 6th, 1954. Sir Roger Bannister ran a mile in 3:59. Until that day no one had ever recorded running a mile under four minutes.

How strong was that unconscious limit? So strong that it only took ***46 days*** for the record to be broken. The unconscious limit had been stripped away, and in only 46 days another runner achieved what only one man had ever achieved before. The sub four minute mile.

The same applies to your exam preparation. Remove your unconscious limits and give your mind the freedom to perform the way it is capable of. Learning to channel self-talk in a positive direction can help you achieve more than you ever imagined.

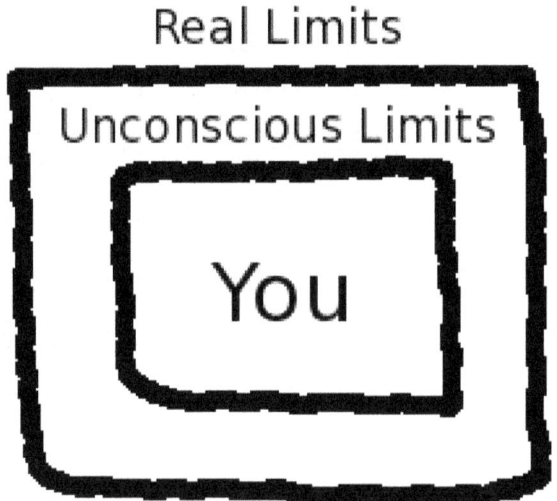

Train Your Mind

In the end, the mind will do what you <u>train</u> it to do. For example, do you ever catch yourself saying subconsciously that you *can't* do something? Of course you have. We all have. That is because we haven't trained our minds to accept the challenge of the task we want to perform.

It is our job to change the way we think. Think positive thoughts. "I CAN do this". "I am the best". "I <u>will</u> pass the exam". Train your mind to think positively and this will reduce your stress level and give you a confident feeling going into the exam.

Do not let others, or your surroundings, dictate your mental state of mind. YOU have the ultimate control and YOU control whether you think positive or negative thoughts.

This takes time and it is something that should be practiced daily. Do not think you can think positive once and everything will occur as you would like it. It just doesn't work that way. Even when you fail, resist the urge to be negative. Everything worthwhile takes some effort. But over time this will work in your favor.

You have to remember you are potentially trying to undo years of "I CAN"T" programming. Years of people telling you "YOU CAN'T" and "NO" and "IT WILL NEVER WORK".

Those are powerful messages built in to your mind. We have all heard them for many years and now is the time to turn it around.

The first "YES I CAN", and "I CAN DO WHATEVER I PUT MY MIND TO" will begin the change. It will start the little snowball rolling down the mountain... and with a little momentum comes massive change!

Self Confidence

Confidence shows in everything you do. From how you look at life to how you treat others. Confident people are people who take action. Confident people are the "doers" in the world. The people who look for ways for things to work rather than look for ways for things to fail.

Confidence is not arrogance. Confidence comes from taking decisive action and not from the outcome of that action. Confident people do not shy away from taking action because they are afraid of a failed outcome. They take action and are undaunted by the prospect of failure.

Arrogance, however, is exactly the opposite. Arrogance does not come from taking action, it comes from the result of the action. Arrogance highlights achievements and hides failures never learning anything from either.

An arrogant person is defined, in their own mind, by both their accomplishments and failures and will shy away from taking action because of the prospect of failure.

Developing Confidence

Confidence is developed through a series of "wins" or "achievements". It is developed through facing your fears and overcoming them. This gives you strength and confidence in your ability to overcome. The more you overcome, the more confident you become.

So how do you build confidence in your ability to pass an exam? Simple.... preparation! Face your fears head on and take action. Prepare every day until you know you are going to pass... there is not doubt!

Review the study material over and over again and build your level of confidence. There is no substitute for hard work and hard work builds confidence.

Have you ever seen a person walk into a room and everyone pays attention? They have a certain confidence about them that radiates form within.

They are not the wealthiest in the room. Nor the most attractive person. But this inner confidence puts them at ease when everyone else may be timid or afraid to step out of their comfort zone.

Confidence and the Exam

Your confidence will have a direct effect on your exam results. If you are confident in your ability to pass the exam it lowers your stress level and opens your mind for clearer thinking. When you project confidence your body reacts differently to circumstances. It gives you the calmness to perform at a high level.

Confidence only comes through preparation. The more you prepare, the more confident you will be in your ability to ace your exam.
This is the type of confidence you must have when you walk into the exam. An undeniable belief that you will pass the exam because of your preparation, determination, and hard work.

Nothing will stand in your way from achieving your goal!

> "YOU GAIN STRENGTH, COURAGE AND CONFIDENCE BY EVERY EXPERIENCE IN WHICH YOU STOP TO LOOK FEAR IN THE FACE. YOU ARE ABLE TO SAY TO YOURSELF, 'I HAVE LIVED THROUGH THIS HORROR. I CAN TAKE THE NEXT THING THAT COMES ALONG.' YOU MUST DO THE THING YOU THINK YOU CANNOT DO."
>
> ELEANOR ROOSEVELT

Sleep and Nutrition

The final piece of the puzzle to reducing stress is proper sleep and nutrition. Your body and mind can only function at its highest level if you give it proper rest and proper nutrition (fuel).

Your body and mind needs time to rest and good food to perform. This is easy to overlook and many times it is the first thing you sacrifice when you are preparing for an exam.

You can do everything else right to reduce stress and prepare for an exam but failing to get proper rest and nutrition could cause it all to go to waste.

Once you think about it you can see why these are essential ingredients (no pun intended) to successful exam preparation.

Sleep

Why is sleep so important? Because it is the only time your body has a chance to recharge.

A good sleep regiment should consist of at least six hours of sleep each night so your body and mind are fresh and ready to go the next morning. Anything less an you will not be fully rested and your performance will suffer because of it.

Stress can also impact sleep patterns to a point that is unhealthy. Stress related sleep disorders are fairly common and can have a major impact on your exam performance.

How many times have you tried to solve work or family related problems well into the night. Sometimes it just cannot be avoided but trying to leave work at work and going to bed with a clear mind will leave you refreshed and ready to tackle the problems of the day when the next day arrives.

To get a better nights sleep try these simple tips to reduce stress and rest up.

1) List problems bothering you with possible solutions before bed.

2) Put work into perspective. When work is over, leave it. Turn it off.

3) Designate cell free time. Even if it is only a half hour or during dinner.

4) Never check work email before bed.

5) Try to simplify one thing each day.

6) Grab a nap if you can. Sleep reduces stress hormones.

7) Laugh! Laughter reduces stress and raises <u>anti-stress</u> hormones making it easier to fall asleep.

8) Owning a pets can significantly lower your heart rate and blood pressure letting you rest longer.

9) Hug a family member. Affection reduces stress and makes it easier to sleep.

10) Take a fifteen minute walk. Exercise is the <u>BEST</u> stress reliever and you will be ready to sleep when the time comes!

These tips can make it easier to get a good nights rest and ready to go in the morning.

Nutrition

Proper nutrition to reduce stress you say? Yes, it's true! Proper nutrition plays a key role in our body's performance and ability to rest.

There is plenty of information about the ties between nutrition and sleep. One of my favorite articles is called "Sleep Deeper with Better Nutrition". It covers a mound of information about protein "super foods" and herbs that will help you get a better nights rest naturally.

Some of the "super foods" are items such as green tea, buffalo, walnuts, sardines, artichokes, kiwis, dark chocolate, cherries, and many others. These foods supply the body with super fuel and burn very efficiently so you don't feel full or tired after eating them.

I prefer making adjustments to diet over prescription drugs or other methods because it is natural and enhances the body's ability to rest.

Food or drink that contain sugar or caffeine can give you a temporary boost but the crash won't help you towards the end of the exam when you typically need it the most so try to avoid these.

What If I Fail?

The most successful people fail all the time! It is a result of taking action. There is no shame in failure, only shame in not getting back up, learning from your mistakes, and trying again.

Golf legend Jack Nicklaus used to welcome a bad golf hole or two each round because the sooner he got them out of the way the sooner he could move on and make the round a great one. He embraced temporary failure as part of being successful.

Truthfully, the more you fail the closer you are to succeeding as long as you learn from your mistakes. Few people succeed without failing many times first. It's a learning process and failure is one of the steps. You can say failure is the downpayment on success and it really is. Chances are good you will fail before you succeed but don't let it define you or hold you back. Expect it and learn from it. If you don't fail it shows you haven't taken action and just sat on the sidelines and that is the worst fate of all.

Overcome your fear of failure and success will be yours. Nothing will stand in your way. Preparation is the key. If you have prepared properly you will not fail. But if you should, embrace it, be accountable for it, and start again with more resolve than ever.

The highway is littered with people who have failed. Everyone fails. The people who win get right back on the horse and start riding again.

> "I HAVE NOT FAILED. I'VE JUST FOUND 10,000 WAYS THAT WON'T WORK."
>
> THOMAS EDISON

Getting Help

Is there a certain section of material that is just not making sense or sinking in? GET HELP! Don't wait or, worse yet, be too shy to ask for help. Search out help as fast as you can. Now is not the time to be shy or hesitate to ask for assistance.

Many teachers and instructors are more than willing to give you a helping hand. That is their profession and most of them generally love to help people. Take advantage of their help if you need it.

REMEMBER, YOU ARE NOT IN THIS ALONE!

Reaching out for help and getting it will give you a feeling of accomplishment and confidence. That confidence will be your friend and something you want to continually build upon as you ready yourself for your exam.

> "ONE IMPORTANT KEY TO SUCCESS IS SELF-CONFIDENCE. AN IMPORTANT KEY TO SELF- CONFIDENCE IS PREPARATION."
>
> ARTHUR ASHE

Common Anatomical Terminology

Anatomy terminology can seem complex and overwhelming when just starting out. Once you familiarize yourself with some of the more common terms it will make your preparation much easier. Just like anything else, it will take practice. Learn and few terms each day and before you know it you will have established a good base to work from.

Take time to familiarize yourself with these terms to make you a better medical coder.

Anatomy Terminology - Number	
Term	**Meaning**
mono-, uni-	one
bi	two
tri	three

Anatomy Terminology - Direction and Position

Term	Meaning
ab-	away from
ad-	toward
ecto-, exo-	outside
endo-	inside
epi-	upon
anterior or ventral	at or near the front surface of the body
posterior or dorsal	at or near the real surface of the body
superior	above
inferior	below
lateral	side
distal	farthest from center
proximal	nearest to center

Anatomy Terminology - Basic Terms

Term	Meaning
abdominal	abdomen
buccal	cheek
cranial	skull
digital	fingers and toes
femoral	thigh
gluteal	buttocks
hallux	great toe
inguinal	groin
lumbar	lowest part of spine
mammary	breast
nasal	nose
occipital	back of head
pectoral	breastbone
thoracic	chest
umbilical	navel
ventral	belly

Anatomy Terminology - Conditions - Prefixes

Term	Meaning
ambi-	both
dys-	bad, painful, difficult
eu-	good, normal
homo-	same
iso-	equal, same
mal-	bad, poor

Anatomy Terminology - Conditions - Suffixes

Term	Meaning
-algia	pain
-emia	blood
-itis	inflammation
-lysis	destruction, breakdown
-oid	like
-opathy	disease of
-pnea	breathing

Anatomy Terminology - Surgical Procedures

Term	Meaning
-centesis	puncture a cavity to remove fluid
-ectomy	surgical removal or excision
-ostomy	a new permanent opening
-otomy	cutting into, incision
-opexy	surgical fixation
-oplasty	surgical repair
-otripsy	crushing or destroying

Medical Terminology Prefix, Root, and Suffixes

Being familiar with Medical Terminology prefixes, roots and suffixes are essential for a medical coder. This illustrates how roots, prefixes, and suffixes are used to denote number or size, direction, color, anatomical locations, as well as other meanings.

Medical Terminology - Prefixes and Roots Denoting Number or Size	
Term	**Meaning**
bi-	two
dipl/o	two, double
hemi-	half
hyper-	over or more than usual
hypo-	under or less than usual
iso-	equal, same
macro-	large
megal/o-	enlargement
micro-	small
mono-	one
multi-	many
nulli-	none
poly-	many
semi-	half, partial
tri-	three
uni-	one

Medical Terminology - Roots Denoting Color

Term	Meaning
chlor/o	green
cyan/o	blue
erythr/o	red
leuk/o	white
melan/o	black
xanth/o	yellow

Medical Terminology - Prefixes and Roots Denoting Relative Direction

Term	Meaning
per-	through
peri-	around
post-	behind, after
poster/o	behind
pre-	before, in front of
pro-	before
retr/o	behind, in back of
sub-	under
super-	beyond
supra-	above
syn-	together
trans-	across
ventr/o	belly

Medical Terminology - Roots Denoting Anatomical Location

Term	Meaning
abdomin/o	abdomen
acr/o	extremity
aden/o	gland
angi/o	vessel
arter/i/o	artery
arthr/o	joint
blast/o	embryo
blephar/o	eyelid
bronch/i/o	bronchus
calcane/o	calaneous
cardi/o	heart
carp/o	carpal, wrist
cephal/o	head
cerebr/o	cerebrum
cheil/o	lip
chol/e	bile, gall
chondr/o	cartilage
cocc/i	coccus
col/o	colon
colp/o	vagina

Medical Terminology - Roots Denoting Anatomical Location

Term	Meaning
condyl/o	condyle
core/o, cor/o	pupil
corne/o	cornea
cost/o	ribs
crani/o	cranium
cycl/o	ciliary body
cyst/o	bladder, sac
cyt/o	cell
dactyl/o	fingers or toes
dent/o	tooth
derm/o	skin
dermat/o	skin
duoden/o	duodenum
enter/o	intestine
esophag/o	esophagus
fibr/o	fiber
gangli/o	ganglion
gastr/o	stomach
gingiv/o	gums
gloss/o	tongue

Medical Terminology - Roots Denoting Anatomical Location

Term	Meaning
gynec/o	women
hem/o, hemat/o	blood
hepat/o	liver
hidr/o	sweat
humer/o	humerus
hydr/o	water
hyster/o	uterus
ile/o	ileum
irid/o, ir/o	iris
ischi/o	ischium
jejun/o	jejunum
kerat/o	cornea
lacrim/o	tear
laryng/o	larynx
lip/o	fat
lith/o	stone, calculus
lumb/o	loin, lumbar area
ment/o	chin
my/o	muscle
myel/o	spinal cord, bone marrow

Medical Terminology - Roots Denoting Anatomical Location

Term	Meaning
nas/o	nose
nephr/o	kidney
neur/o	nerve
omphal/o	umbilicus, navel
onych/o	nail
oophor/o	ovary
opthalm/o	eye
orchid/o	testicles
oste/o	bone
ot/o	ear
pancreat/o	pancreas
pely/i	pelvis
peps/o/ia	digestion
phalang/o	phalange
pharyng/o	pharynx
phas/o	speech
phleb/o	veins
pleur/o	pleura
pne/o	air, breathing
pneum/o, pneumono	lung

Medical Terminology - Roots Denoting Anatomical Location

Term	Meaning
pod/o	foot
proct/o	rectum, anus
psych/o	mind
pub/o	pubis
py/o	pus
pyel/o	kidney
rect/o	rectum
ren/o	kidney
retin/o	retina
rhin/o	nose
salping/o	fallopian tube
scler/o	sclera
spermat/o	sperm
splen/o	spleen
stern/o	sternum, breastbone
stomat/o	mouth
thorac/o	thorax, chest
trache/o	trachea
traumat/o	tramua
tympan/o	eardrum

Medical Terminology - Roots Denoting Anatomical Location

Term	Meaning
ur/o	urine
ureter/o	ureter
urethr/o	urethra
vas/o	vessel
viscer/o	gut, contents of the abdomen

Medical Terminology - Other Prefixes

Term	Meaning
a-, an-	without
anti-	against
auto-	self
brady-	slow
con-	with
contra-	against
dis-	free of
dys-	difficult or without pain
mal-	bad, poor
neo-	new
syn-	together
tachy-	fast

Medical Terminology - Other Roots

Term	Meaning
necr/o	dead
noct/i	night
par/o	bear
phag/o	eat
phil/o	attraction
plast/o	repair, formation
pyr/o	fire, fever
scler/o	tough, hard
sinistr/o	left
syphil/o	syphilis
therap/o	treatment
therm/o	heat
thromb/o	thrombosis
troph/o	development

Medical Terminology - Other Suffixes

Term	Meaning
algia	pain
ar	pertaining to
centesis	puncture
clysis	irrigation
ectasia	dilatation, dilation
ectomy	excision
emes/is	vomiting
emia	blood
esthesia	feelings
genesis, gen/o	development, formation, beginning
gnosis	know
ia	noun ending
ia, ic	pertaining to
it is	inflammation
manual	hand
meter	measuring instrument
oid	resembling
ologist	one who studies
ology	study of
oma	tumor

Medical Terminology - Other Suffixes

Term	Meaning
opia	vision
orrhagia	hemorrhage
orrhaphy	suture
orrhea	flow
orrhexis	rupture
osis	condition of
ostomy	new opening
otomy	incision
pedal	foot
pexy	fixing, fixation
phob/ia	fear
plasm	growth
plegia, plegic	paralysis
ptosis	drooping
scope, scopy	examining, looking at
spasm	twitching
sperm	sperm
stasis	slow, stop
tome	instrument
tripsy	crushing

Notes

Notes

Scoring Sheets
(tear out for easy use)

#					#					#				
1)	A	B	C	D	26)	A	B	C	D	53)	A	B	C	D
2)	A	B	C	D	27)	A	B	C	D	54)	A	B	C	D
3)	A	B	C	D	28)	A	B	C	D	55)	A	B	C	D
4)	A	B	C	D	29)	A	B	C	D	56)	A	B	C	D
5)	A	B	C	D	30)	A	B	C	D	57)	A	B	C	D
6)	A	B	C	D	31)	A	B	C	D	58)	A	B	C	D
7)	A	B	C	D	32)	A	B	C	D	59)	A	B	C	D
8)	A	B	C	D	33)	A	B	C	D	60)	A	B	C	D
9)	A	B	C	D	34)	A	B	C	D	61)	A	B	C	D
10)	A	B	C	D	35)	A	B	C	D	62)	A	B	C	D
11)	A	B	C	D	36)	A	B	C	D	63)	A	B	C	D
12)	A	B	C	D	37)	A	B	C	D	64)	A	B	C	D
13)	A	B	C	D	38)	A	B	C	D	65)	A	B	C	D
14)	A	B	C	D	39)	A	B	C	D	66)	A	B	C	D
15)	A	B	C	D	40)	A	B	C	D	67)	A	B	C	D
16)	A	B	C	D	41)	A	B	C	D	68)	A	B	C	D
17)	A	B	C	D	42)	A	B	C	D	69)	A	B	C	D
18)	A	B	C	D	43)	A	B	C	D	70)	A	B	C	D
19)	A	B	C	D	44)	A	B	C	D	71)	A	B	C	D
20)	A	B	C	D	45)	A	B	C	D	72)	A	B	C	D
21)	A	B	C	D	46)	A	B	C	D	73)	A	B	C	D
22)	A	B	C	D	47)	A	B	C	D	74)	A	B	C	D
23)	A	B	C	D	48)	A	B	C	D	75)	A	B	C	D
24)	A	B	C	D	49)	A	B	C	D	76)	A	B	C	D
25)	A	B	C	D	50)	A	B	C	D	77)	A	B	C	D
					51)	A	B	C	D	78)	A	B	C	D
					52)	A	B	C	D	79)	A	B	C	D

80)	A	B	C	D	107)	A	B	C	D	134)	A	B	C	D
81)	A	B	C	D	108)	A	B	C	D	135)	A	B	C	D
82)	A	B	C	D	109)	A	B	C	D	136)	A	B	C	D
83)	A	B	C	D	110)	A	B	C	D	137)	A	B	C	D
84)	A	B	C	D	111)	A	B	C	D	138)	A	B	C	D
85)	A	B	C	D	112)	A	B	C	D	139)	A	B	C	D
86)	A	B	C	D	113)	A	B	C	D	140)	A	B	C	D
87)	A	B	C	D	114)	A	B	C	D	141)	A	B	C	D
88)	A	B	C	D	115)	A	B	C	D	142)	A	B	C	D
89)	A	B	C	D	116)	A	B	C	D	143)	A	B	C	D
90)	A	B	C	D	117)	A	B	C	D	144)	A	B	C	D
91)	A	B	C	D	118)	A	B	C	D	145)	A	B	C	D
92)	A	B	C	D	119)	A	B	C	D	146)	A	B	C	D
93)	A	B	C	D	120)	A	B	C	D	147)	A	B	C	D
94)	A	B	C	D	121)	A	B	C	D	148)	A	B	C	D
95)	A	B	C	D	122)	A	B	C	D	149)	A	B	C	D
96)	A	B	C	D	123)	A	B	C	D	150)	A	B	C	D
97)	A	B	C	D	124)	A	B	C	D					
98)	A	B	C	D	125)	A	B	C	D					
99)	A	B	C	D	126)	A	B	C	D					
100)	A	B	C	D	127)	A	B	C	D					
101)	A	B	C	D	128)	A	B	C	D					
102)	A	B	C	D	129)	A	B	C	D					
103)	A	B	C	D	130)	A	B	C	D					
104)	A	B	C	D	131)	A	B	C	D					
105)	A	B	C	D	132)	A	B	C	D					
106)	A	B	C	D	133)	A	B	C	D					

Scoring Sheet 2
(tear out for easy use)

#					#					#				
1)	A	B	C	D	27)	A	B	C	D	54)	A	B	C	D
2)	A	B	C	D	28)	A	B	C	D	55)	A	B	C	D
3)	A	B	C	D	29)	A	B	C	D	56)	A	B	C	D
4)	A	B	C	D	30)	A	B	C	D	57)	A	B	C	D
5)	A	B	C	D	31)	A	B	C	D	58)	A	B	C	D
6)	A	B	C	D	32)	A	B	C	D	59)	A	B	C	D
7)	A	B	C	D	33)	A	B	C	D	60)	A	B	C	D
8)	A	B	C	D	34)	A	B	C	D	61)	A	B	C	D
9)	A	B	C	D	35)	A	B	C	D	62)	A	B	C	D
10)	A	B	C	D	36)	A	B	C	D	63)	A	B	C	D
11)	A	B	C	D	37)	A	B	C	D	64)	A	B	C	D
12)	A	B	C	D	38)	A	B	C	D	65)	A	B	C	D
13)	A	B	C	D	39)	A	B	C	D	66)	A	B	C	D
14)	A	B	C	D	40)	A	B	C	D	67)	A	B	C	D
15)	A	B	C	D	41)	A	B	C	D	68)	A	B	C	D
16)	A	B	C	D	42)	A	B	C	D	69)	A	B	C	D
17)	A	B	C	D	43)	A	B	C	D	70)	A	B	C	D
18)	A	B	C	D	44)	A	B	C	D	71)	A	B	C	D
19)	A	B	C	D	45)	A	B	C	D	72)	A	B	C	D
20)	A	B	C	D	46)	A	B	C	D	73)	A	B	C	D
21)	A	B	C	D	47)	A	B	C	D	74)	A	B	C	D
22)	A	B	C	D	48)	A	B	C	D	75)	A	B	C	D
23)	A	B	C	D	49)	A	B	C	D	76)	A	B	C	D
24)	A	B	C	D	50)	A	B	C	D	77)	A	B	C	D
25)	A	B	C	D	51)	A	B	C	D	78)	A	B	C	D
26)	A	B	C	D	52)	A	B	C	D	79)	A	B	C	D
					53)	A	B	C	D	80)	A	B	C	D

PROPERTY OF MEDICAL CODING PRO UNAUTHORIZED DISTRIBUTION PROHIBITED SINGLE COPY LICENSE

81)	A	B	C	D	108)	A	B	C	D	135)	A	B	C	D
82)	A	B	C	D	109)	A	B	C	D	136)	A	B	C	D
83)	A	B	C	D	110)	A	B	C	D	137)	A	B	C	D
84)	A	B	C	D	111)	A	B	C	D	138)	A	B	C	D
85)	A	B	C	D	112)	A	B	C	D	139)	A	B	C	D
86)	A	B	C	D	113)	A	B	C	D	140)	A	B	C	D
87)	A	B	C	D	114)	A	B	C	D	141)	A	B	C	D
88)	A	B	C	D	115)	A	B	C	D	142)	A	B	C	D
89)	A	B	C	D	116)	A	B	C	D	143)	A	B	C	D
90)	A	B	C	D	117)	A	B	C	D	144)	A	B	C	D
91)	A	B	C	D	118)	A	B	C	D	145)	A	B	C	D
92)	A	B	C	D	119)	A	B	C	D	146)	A	B	C	D
93)	A	B	C	D	120)	A	B	C	D	147)	A	B	C	D
94)	A	B	C	D	121)	A	B	C	D	148)	A	B	C	D
95)	A	B	C	D	122)	A	B	C	D	149)	A	B	C	D
96)	A	B	C	D	123)	A	B	C	D	150)	A	B	C	D
97)	A	B	C	D	124)	A	B	C	D					
98)	A	B	C	D	125)	A	B	C	D					
99)	A	B	C	D	126)	A	B	C	D					
100)	A	B	C	D	127)	A	B	C	D					
101)	A	B	C	D	128)	A	B	C	D					
102)	A	B	C	D	129)	A	B	C	D					
103)	A	B	C	D	130)	A	B	C	D					
104)	A	B	C	D	131)	A	B	C	D					
105)	A	B	C	D	132)	A	B	C	D					
106)	A	B	C	D	133)	A	B	C	D					
107)	A	B	C	D	134)	A	B	C	D					

Scoring Sheet 3
(tear out for easy use)

#					#					#				
1)	A	B	C	D	26)	A	B	C	D	53)	A	B	C	D
2)	A	B	C	D	27)	A	B	C	D	54)	A	B	C	D
3)	A	B	C	D	28)	A	B	C	D	55)	A	B	C	D
4)	A	B	C	D	29)	A	B	C	D	56)	A	B	C	D
5)	A	B	C	D	30)	A	B	C	D	57)	A	B	C	D
6)	A	B	C	D	31)	A	B	C	D	58)	A	B	C	D
7)	A	B	C	D	32)	A	B	C	D	59)	A	B	C	D
8)	A	B	C	D	33)	A	B	C	D	60)	A	B	C	D
9)	A	B	C	D	34)	A	B	C	D	61)	A	B	C	D
10)	A	B	C	D	35)	A	B	C	D	62)	A	B	C	D
11)	A	B	C	D	36)	A	B	C	D	63)	A	B	C	D
12)	A	B	C	D	37)	A	B	C	D	64)	A	B	C	D
13)	A	B	C	D	38)	A	B	C	D	65)	A	B	C	D
14)	A	B	C	D	39)	A	B	C	D	66)	A	B	C	D
15)	A	B	C	D	40)	A	B	C	D	67)	A	B	C	D
16)	A	B	C	D	41)	A	B	C	D	68)	A	B	C	D
17)	A	B	C	D	42)	A	B	C	D	69)	A	B	C	D
18)	A	B	C	D	43)	A	B	C	D	70)	A	B	C	D
19)	A	B	C	D	44)	A	B	C	D	71)	A	B	C	D
20)	A	B	C	D	45)	A	B	C	D	72)	A	B	C	D
21)	A	B	C	D	46)	A	B	C	D	73)	A	B	C	D
22)	A	B	C	D	47)	A	B	C	D	74)	A	B	C	D
23)	A	B	C	D	48)	A	B	C	D	75)	A	B	C	D
24)	A	B	C	D	49)	A	B	C	D	76)	A	B	C	D
25)	A	B	C	D	50)	A	B	C	D	77)	A	B	C	D
					51)	A	B	C	D	78)	A	B	C	D
					52)	A	B	C	D	79)	A	B	C	D

80)	A	B	C	D	107)	A	B	C	D	134)	A	B	C	D
81)	A	B	C	D	108)	A	B	C	D	135)	A	B	C	D
82)	A	B	C	D	109)	A	B	C	D	136)	A	B	C	D
83)	A	B	C	D	110)	A	B	C	D	137)	A	B	C	D
84)	A	B	C	D	111)	A	B	C	D	138)	A	B	C	D
85)	A	B	C	D	112)	A	B	C	D	139)	A	B	C	D
86)	A	B	C	D	113)	A	B	C	D	140)	A	B	C	D
87)	A	B	C	D	114)	A	B	C	D	141)	A	B	C	D
88)	A	B	C	D	115)	A	B	C	D	142)	A	B	C	D
89)	A	B	C	D	116)	A	B	C	D	143)	A	B	C	D
90)	A	B	C	D	117)	A	B	C	D	144)	A	B	C	D
91)	A	B	C	D	118)	A	B	C	D	145)	A	B	C	D
92)	A	B	C	D	119)	A	B	C	D	146)	A	B	C	D
93)	A	B	C	D	120)	A	B	C	D	147)	A	B	C	D
94)	A	B	C	D	121)	A	B	C	D	148)	A	B	C	D
95)	A	B	C	D	122)	A	B	C	D	149)	A	B	C	D
96)	A	B	C	D	123)	A	B	C	D	150)	A	B	C	D
97)	A	B	C	D	124)	A	B	C	D					
98)	A	B	C	D	125)	A	B	C	D	XXXXXXXXXXXXXX				
99)	A	B	C	D	126)	A	B	C	D	XXXXXXXXXXXXXX				
100)	A	B	C	D	127)	A	B	C	D	XXXXXXXXXXXXXX				
101)	A	B	C	D	128)	A	B	C	D	XXXXXXXXXXXXXX				
102)	A	B	C	D	129)	A	B	C	D					
103)	A	B	C	D	130)	A	B	C	D					
104)	A	B	C	D	131)	A	B	C	D					
105)	A	B	C	D	132)	A	B	C	D					
106)	A	B	C	D	133)	A	B	C	D					

Scoring Sheet 4
(tear out for easy use)

#					#					#				
1)	A	B	C	D	26)	A	B	C	D	53)	A	B	C	D
2)	A	B	C	D	27)	A	B	C	D	54)	A	B	C	D
3)	A	B	C	D	28)	A	B	C	D	55)	A	B	C	D
4)	A	B	C	D	29)	A	B	C	D	56)	A	B	C	D
5)	A	B	C	D	30)	A	B	C	D	57)	A	B	C	D
6)	A	B	C	D	31)	A	B	C	D	58)	A	B	C	D
7)	A	B	C	D	32)	A	B	C	D	59)	A	B	C	D
8)	A	B	C	D	33)	A	B	C	D	60)	A	B	C	D
9)	A	B	C	D	34)	A	B	C	D	61)	A	B	C	D
10)	A	B	C	D	35)	A	B	C	D	62)	A	B	C	D
11)	A	B	C	D	36)	A	B	C	D	63)	A	B	C	D
12)	A	B	C	D	37)	A	B	C	D	64)	A	B	C	D
13)	A	B	C	D	38)	A	B	C	D	65)	A	B	C	D
14)	A	B	C	D	39)	A	B	C	D	66)	A	B	C	D
15)	A	B	C	D	40)	A	B	C	D	67)	A	B	C	D
16)	A	B	C	D	41)	A	B	C	D	68)	A	B	C	D
17)	A	B	C	D	42)	A	B	C	D	69)	A	B	C	D
18)	A	B	C	D	43)	A	B	C	D	70)	A	B	C	D
19)	A	B	C	D	44)	A	B	C	D	71)	A	B	C	D
20)	A	B	C	D	45)	A	B	C	D	72)	A	B	C	D
21)	A	B	C	D	46)	A	B	C	D	73)	A	B	C	D
22)	A	B	C	D	47)	A	B	C	D	74)	A	B	C	D
23)	A	B	C	D	48)	A	B	C	D	75)	A	B	C	D
24)	A	B	C	D	49)	A	B	C	D	76)	A	B	C	D
25)	A	B	C	D	50)	A	B	C	D	77)	A	B	C	D
					51)	A	B	C	D	78)	A	B	C	D
					52)	A	B	C	D	79)	A	B	C	D

80)	A	B	C	D	107)	A	B	C	D	134)	A	B	C	D
81)	A	B	C	D	108)	A	B	C	D	135)	A	B	C	D
82)	A	B	C	D	109)	A	B	C	D	136)	A	B	C	D
83)	A	B	C	D	110)	A	B	C	D	137)	A	B	C	D
84)	A	B	C	D	111)	A	B	C	D	138)	A	B	C	D
85)	A	B	C	D	112)	A	B	C	D	139)	A	B	C	D
86)	A	B	C	D	113)	A	B	C	D	140)	A	B	C	D
87)	A	B	C	D	114)	A	B	C	D	141)	A	B	C	D
88)	A	B	C	D	115)	A	B	C	D	142)	A	B	C	D
89)	A	B	C	D	116)	A	B	C	D	143)	A	B	C	D
90)	A	B	C	D	117)	A	B	C	D	144)	A	B	C	D
91)	A	B	C	D	118)	A	B	C	D	145)	A	B	C	D
92)	A	B	C	D	119)	A	B	C	D	146)	A	B	C	D
93)	A	B	C	D	120)	A	B	C	D	147)	A	B	C	D
94)	A	B	C	D	121)	A	B	C	D	148)	A	B	C	D
95)	A	B	C	D	122)	A	B	C	D	149)	A	B	C	D
96)	A	B	C	D	123)	A	B	C	D	150)	A	B	C	D
97)	A	B	C	D	124)	A	B	C	D					
98)	A	B	C	D	125)	A	B	C	D	XXXXXXXXXXXXXXX
99)	A	B	C	D	126)	A	B	C	D	XXXXXXXXXXXXXXX
100)	A	B	C	D	127)	A	B	C	D	XXXXXXXXXXXXXXX
101)	A	B	C	D	128)	A	B	C	D	XXXXXXXXXXXXXXX
102)	A	B	C	D	129)	A	B	C	D					
103)	A	B	C	D	130)	A	B	C	D					
104)	A	B	C	D	131)	A	B	C	D					
105)	A	B	C	D	132)	A	B	C	D					
106)	A	B	C	D	133)	A	B	C	D					

Scoring Sheet 5
(tear out for easy use)

#					#					#				
1)	A	B	C	D	26)	A	B	C	D	53)	A	B	C	D
2)	A	B	C	D	27)	A	B	C	D	54)	A	B	C	D
3)	A	B	C	D	28)	A	B	C	D	55)	A	B	C	D
4)	A	B	C	D	29)	A	B	C	D	56)	A	B	C	D
5)	A	B	C	D	30)	A	B	C	D	57)	A	B	C	D
6)	A	B	C	D	31)	A	B	C	D	58)	A	B	C	D
7)	A	B	C	D	32)	A	B	C	D	59)	A	B	C	D
8)	A	B	C	D	33)	A	B	C	D	60)	A	B	C	D
9)	A	B	C	D	34)	A	B	C	D	61)	A	B	C	D
10)	A	B	C	D	35)	A	B	C	D	62)	A	B	C	D
11)	A	B	C	D	36)	A	B	C	D	63)	A	B	C	D
12)	A	B	C	D	37)	A	B	C	D	64)	A	B	C	D
13)	A	B	C	D	38)	A	B	C	D	65)	A	B	C	D
14)	A	B	C	D	39)	A	B	C	D	66)	A	B	C	D
15)	A	B	C	D	40)	A	B	C	D	67)	A	B	C	D
16)	A	B	C	D	41)	A	B	C	D	68)	A	B	C	D
17)	A	B	C	D	42)	A	B	C	D	69)	A	B	C	D
18)	A	B	C	D	43)	A	B	C	D	70)	A	B	C	D
19)	A	B	C	D	44)	A	B	C	D	71)	A	B	C	D
20)	A	B	C	D	45)	A	B	C	D	72)	A	B	C	D
21)	A	B	C	D	46)	A	B	C	D	73)	A	B	C	D
22)	A	B	C	D	47)	A	B	C	D	74)	A	B	C	D
23)	A	B	C	D	48)	A	B	C	D	75)	A	B	C	D
24)	A	B	C	D	49)	A	B	C	D	76)	A	B	C	D
25)	A	B	C	D	50)	A	B	C	D	77)	A	B	C	D
					51)	A	B	C	D	78)	A	B	C	D
					52)	A	B	C	D	79)	A	B	C	D

80)	A	B	C	D	107)	A	B	C	D	134)	A	B	C	D
81)	A	B	C	D	108)	A	B	C	D	135)	A	B	C	D
82)	A	B	C	D	109)	A	B	C	D	136)	A	B	C	D
83)	A	B	C	D	110)	A	B	C	D	137)	A	B	C	D
84)	A	B	C	D	111)	A	B	C	D	138)	A	B	C	D
85)	A	B	C	D	112)	A	B	C	D	139)	A	B	C	D
86)	A	B	C	D	113)	A	B	C	D	140)	A	B	C	D
87)	A	B	C	D	114)	A	B	C	D	141)	A	B	C	D
88)	A	B	C	D	115)	A	B	C	D	142)	A	B	C	D
89)	A	B	C	D	116)	A	B	C	D	143)	A	B	C	D
90)	A	B	C	D	117)	A	B	C	D	144)	A	B	C	D
91)	A	B	C	D	118)	A	B	C	D	145)	A	B	C	D
92)	A	B	C	D	119)	A	B	C	D	146)	A	B	C	D
93)	A	B	C	D	120)	A	B	C	D	147)	A	B	C	D
94)	A	B	C	D	121)	A	B	C	D	148)	A	B	C	D
95)	A	B	C	D	122)	A	B	C	D	149)	A	B	C	D
96)	A	B	C	D	123)	A	B	C	D	150)	A	B	C	D
97)	A	B	C	D	124)	A	B	C	D					
98)	A	B	C	D	125)	A	B	C	D	XXXXXXXXXXXXXXX				
99)	A	B	C	D	126)	A	B	C	D	XXXXXXXXXXXXXXX				
100)	A	B	C	D	127)	A	B	C	D	XXXXXXXXXXXXXXX				
101)	A	B	C	D	128)	A	B	C	D	XXXXXXXXXXXXXXX				
102)	A	B	C	D	129)	A	B	C	D					
103)	A	B	C	D	130)	A	B	C	D					
104)	A	B	C	D	131)	A	B	C	D					
105)	A	B	C	D	132)	A	B	C	D					
106)	A	B	C	D	133)	A	B	C	D					

Scoring Sheet 6
(tear out for easy use)

#					#					#				
1)	A	B	C	D	26)	A	B	C	D	53)	A	B	C	D
2)	A	B	C	D	27)	A	B	C	D	54)	A	B	C	D
3)	A	B	C	D	28)	A	B	C	D	55)	A	B	C	D
4)	A	B	C	D	29)	A	B	C	D	56)	A	B	C	D
5)	A	B	C	D	30)	A	B	C	D	57)	A	B	C	D
6)	A	B	C	D	31)	A	B	C	D	58)	A	B	C	D
7)	A	B	C	D	32)	A	B	C	D	59)	A	B	C	D
8)	A	B	C	D	33)	A	B	C	D	60)	A	B	C	D
9)	A	B	C	D	34)	A	B	C	D	61)	A	B	C	D
10)	A	B	C	D	35)	A	B	C	D	62)	A	B	C	D
11)	A	B	C	D	36)	A	B	C	D	63)	A	B	C	D
12)	A	B	C	D	37)	A	B	C	D	64)	A	B	C	D
13)	A	B	C	D	38)	A	B	C	D	65)	A	B	C	D
14)	A	B	C	D	39)	A	B	C	D	66)	A	B	C	D
15)	A	B	C	D	40)	A	B	C	D	67)	A	B	C	D
16)	A	B	C	D	41)	A	B	C	D	68)	A	B	C	D
17)	A	B	C	D	42)	A	B	C	D	69)	A	B	C	D
18)	A	B	C	D	43)	A	B	C	D	70)	A	B	C	D
19)	A	B	C	D	44)	A	B	C	D	71)	A	B	C	D
20)	A	B	C	D	45)	A	B	C	D	72)	A	B	C	D
21)	A	B	C	D	46)	A	B	C	D	73)	A	B	C	D
22)	A	B	C	D	47)	A	B	C	D	74)	A	B	C	D
23)	A	B	C	D	48)	A	B	C	D	75)	A	B	C	D
24)	A	B	C	D	49)	A	B	C	D	76)	A	B	C	D
25)	A	B	C	D	50)	A	B	C	D	77)	A	B	C	D
					51)	A	B	C	D	78)	A	B	C	D
					52)	A	B	C	D	79)	A	B	C	D

80)	A	B	C	D	107)	A	B	C	D	134)	A	B	C	D
81)	A	B	C	D	108)	A	B	C	D	135)	A	B	C	D
82)	A	B	C	D	109)	A	B	C	D	136)	A	B	C	D
83)	A	B	C	D	110)	A	B	C	D	137)	A	B	C	D
84)	A	B	C	D	111)	A	B	C	D	138)	A	B	C	D
85)	A	B	C	D	112)	A	B	C	D	139)	A	B	C	D
86)	A	B	C	D	113)	A	B	C	D	140)	A	B	C	D
87)	A	B	C	D	114)	A	B	C	D	141)	A	B	C	D
88)	A	B	C	D	115)	A	B	C	D	142)	A	B	C	D
89)	A	B	C	D	116)	A	B	C	D	143)	A	B	C	D
90)	A	B	C	D	117)	A	B	C	D	144)	A	B	C	D
91)	A	B	C	D	118)	A	B	C	D	145)	A	B	C	D
92)	A	B	C	D	119)	A	B	C	D	146)	A	B	C	D
93)	A	B	C	D	120)	A	B	C	D	147)	A	B	C	D
94)	A	B	C	D	121)	A	B	C	D	148)	A	B	C	D
95)	A	B	C	D	122)	A	B	C	D	149)	A	B	C	D
96)	A	B	C	D	123)	A	B	C	D	150)	A	B	C	D
97)	A	B	C	D	124)	A	B	C	D					
98)	A	B	C	D	125)	A	B	C	D	XXXXXXXXXXXXXXX
99)	A	B	C	D	126)	A	B	C	D	XXXXXXXXXXXXXXX
100)	A	B	C	D	127)	A	B	C	D	XXXXXXXXXXXXXXX
101)	A	B	C	D	128)	A	B	C	D	XXXXXXXXXXXXXXX
102)	A	B	C	D	129)	A	B	C	D					
103)	A	B	C	D	130)	A	B	C	D					
104)	A	B	C	D	131)	A	B	C	D					
105)	A	B	C	D	132)	A	B	C	D					
106)	A	B	C	D	133)	A	B	C	D					

Scoring Sheet 7
(tear out for easy use)

#					#					#				
1)	A	B	C	D	26)	A	B	C	D	53)	A	B	C	D
2)	A	B	C	D	27)	A	B	C	D	54)	A	B	C	D
3)	A	B	C	D	28)	A	B	C	D	55)	A	B	C	D
4)	A	B	C	D	29)	A	B	C	D	56)	A	B	C	D
5)	A	B	C	D	30)	A	B	C	D	57)	A	B	C	D
6)	A	B	C	D	31)	A	B	C	D	58)	A	B	C	D
7)	A	B	C	D	32)	A	B	C	D	59)	A	B	C	D
8)	A	B	C	D	33)	A	B	C	D	60)	A	B	C	D
9)	A	B	C	D	34)	A	B	C	D	61)	A	B	C	D
10)	A	B	C	D	35)	A	B	C	D	62)	A	B	C	D
11)	A	B	C	D	36)	A	B	C	D	63)	A	B	C	D
12)	A	B	C	D	37)	A	B	C	D	64)	A	B	C	D
13)	A	B	C	D	38)	A	B	C	D	65)	A	B	C	D
14)	A	B	C	D	39)	A	B	C	D	66)	A	B	C	D
15)	A	B	C	D	40)	A	B	C	D	67)	A	B	C	D
16)	A	B	C	D	41)	A	B	C	D	68)	A	B	C	D
17)	A	B	C	D	42)	A	B	C	D	69)	A	B	C	D
18)	A	B	C	D	43)	A	B	C	D	70)	A	B	C	D
19)	A	B	C	D	44)	A	B	C	D	71)	A	B	C	D
20)	A	B	C	D	45)	A	B	C	D	72)	A	B	C	D
21)	A	B	C	D	46)	A	B	C	D	73)	A	B	C	D
22)	A	B	C	D	47)	A	B	C	D	74)	A	B	C	D
23)	A	B	C	D	48)	A	B	C	D	75)	A	B	C	D
24)	A	B	C	D	49)	A	B	C	D	76)	A	B	C	D
25)	A	B	C	D	50)	A	B	C	D	77)	A	B	C	D
					51)	A	B	C	D	78)	A	B	C	D
					52)	A	B	C	D	79)	A	B	C	D

PROPERTY OF MEDICAL CODING PRO UNAUTHORIZED DISTRIBUTION PROHIBITED SINGLE COPY LICENSE

80)	A	B	C	D	107)	A	B	C	D	134)	A	B	C	D
81)	A	B	C	D	108)	A	B	C	D	135)	A	B	C	D
82)	A	B	C	D	109)	A	B	C	D	136)	A	B	C	D
83)	A	B	C	D	110)	A	B	C	D	137)	A	B	C	D
84)	A	B	C	D	111)	A	B	C	D	138)	A	B	C	D
85)	A	B	C	D	112)	A	B	C	D	139)	A	B	C	D
86)	A	B	C	D	113)	A	B	C	D	140)	A	B	C	D
87)	A	B	C	D	114)	A	B	C	D	141)	A	B	C	D
88)	A	B	C	D	115)	A	B	C	D	142)	A	B	C	D
89)	A	B	C	D	116)	A	B	C	D	143)	A	B	C	D
90)	A	B	C	D	117)	A	B	C	D	144)	A	B	C	D
91)	A	B	C	D	118)	A	B	C	D	145)	A	B	C	D
92)	A	B	C	D	119)	A	B	C	D	146)	A	B	C	D
93)	A	B	C	D	120)	A	B	C	D	147)	A	B	C	D
94)	A	B	C	D	121)	A	B	C	D	148)	A	B	C	D
95)	A	B	C	D	122)	A	B	C	D	149)	A	B	C	D
96)	A	B	C	D	123)	A	B	C	D	150)	A	B	C	D
97)	A	B	C	D	124)	A	B	C	D					
98)	A	B	C	D	125)	A	B	C	D					
99)	A	B	C	D	126)	A	B	C	D					
100)	A	B	C	D	127)	A	B	C	D					
101)	A	B	C	D	128)	A	B	C	D					
102)	A	B	C	D	129)	A	B	C	D					
103)	A	B	C	D	130)	A	B	C	D					
104)	A	B	C	D	131)	A	B	C	D					
105)	A	B	C	D	132)	A	B	C	D					
106)	A	B	C	D	133)	A	B	C	D					

Scoring Sheet 8
(tear out for easy use)

#					#					#				
1)	A	B	C	D	26)	A	B	C	D	53)	A	B	C	D
2)	A	B	C	D	27)	A	B	C	D	54)	A	B	C	D
3)	A	B	C	D	28)	A	B	C	D	55)	A	B	C	D
4)	A	B	C	D	29)	A	B	C	D	56)	A	B	C	D
5)	A	B	C	D	30)	A	B	C	D	57)	A	B	C	D
6)	A	B	C	D	31)	A	B	C	D	58)	A	B	C	D
7)	A	B	C	D	32)	A	B	C	D	59)	A	B	C	D
8)	A	B	C	D	33)	A	B	C	D	60)	A	B	C	D
9)	A	B	C	D	34)	A	B	C	D	61)	A	B	C	D
10)	A	B	C	D	35)	A	B	C	D	62)	A	B	C	D
11)	A	B	C	D	36)	A	B	C	D	63)	A	B	C	D
12)	A	B	C	D	37)	A	B	C	D	64)	A	B	C	D
13)	A	B	C	D	38)	A	B	C	D	65)	A	B	C	D
14)	A	B	C	D	39)	A	B	C	D	66)	A	B	C	D
15)	A	B	C	D	40)	A	B	C	D	67)	A	B	C	D
16)	A	B	C	D	41)	A	B	C	D	68)	A	B	C	D
17)	A	B	C	D	42)	A	B	C	D	69)	A	B	C	D
18)	A	B	C	D	43)	A	B	C	D	70)	A	B	C	D
19)	A	B	C	D	44)	A	B	C	D	71)	A	B	C	D
20)	A	B	C	D	45)	A	B	C	D	72)	A	B	C	D
21)	A	B	C	D	46)	A	B	C	D	73)	A	B	C	D
22)	A	B	C	D	47)	A	B	C	D	74)	A	B	C	D
23)	A	B	C	D	48)	A	B	C	D	75)	A	B	C	D
24)	A	B	C	D	49)	A	B	C	D	76)	A	B	C	D
25)	A	B	C	D	50)	A	B	C	D	77)	A	B	C	D
					51)	A	B	C	D	78)	A	B	C	D
					52)	A	B	C	D	79)	A	B	C	D

PROPERTY OF MEDICAL CODING PRO UNAUTHORIZED DISTRIBUTION PROHIBITED SINGLE COPY LICENSE

80)	A	B	C	D	107)	A	B	C	D	134)	A	B	C	D
81)	A	B	C	D	108)	A	B	C	D	135)	A	B	C	D
82)	A	B	C	D	109)	A	B	C	D	136)	A	B	C	D
83)	A	B	C	D	110)	A	B	C	D	137)	A	B	C	D
84)	A	B	C	D	111)	A	B	C	D	138)	A	B	C	D
85)	A	B	C	D	112)	A	B	C	D	139)	A	B	C	D
86)	A	B	C	D	113)	A	B	C	D	140)	A	B	C	D
87)	A	B	C	D	114)	A	B	C	D	141)	A	B	C	D
88)	A	B	C	D	115)	A	B	C	D	142)	A	B	C	D
89)	A	B	C	D	116)	A	B	C	D	143)	A	B	C	D
90)	A	B	C	D	117)	A	B	C	D	144)	A	B	C	D
91)	A	B	C	D	118)	A	B	C	D	145)	A	B	C	D
92)	A	B	C	D	119)	A	B	C	D	146)	A	B	C	D
93)	A	B	C	D	120)	A	B	C	D	147)	A	B	C	D
94)	A	B	C	D	121)	A	B	C	D	148)	A	B	C	D
95)	A	B	C	D	122)	A	B	C	D	149)	A	B	C	D
96)	A	B	C	D	123)	A	B	C	D	150)	A	B	C	D
97)	A	B	C	D	124)	A	B	C	D					
98)	A	B	C	D	125)	A	B	C	D	XXXXXXXXXXXXXX
99)	A	B	C	D	126)	A	B	C	D	XXXXXXXXXXXXXX
100)	A	B	C	D	127)	A	B	C	D	XXXXXXXXXXXXXX
101)	A	B	C	D	128)	A	B	C	D	XXXXXXXXXXXXXX
102)	A	B	C	D	129)	A	B	C	D					
103)	A	B	C	D	130)	A	B	C	D					
104)	A	B	C	D	131)	A	B	C	D					
105)	A	B	C	D	132)	A	B	C	D					
106)	A	B	C	D	133)	A	B	C	D					

Scoring Sheet 9
(tear out for easy use)

#					#					#				
1)	A	B	C	D	26)	A	B	C	D	53)	A	B	C	D
2)	A	B	C	D	27)	A	B	C	D	54)	A	B	C	D
3)	A	B	C	D	28)	A	B	C	D	55)	A	B	C	D
4)	A	B	C	D	29)	A	B	C	D	56)	A	B	C	D
5)	A	B	C	D	30)	A	B	C	D	57)	A	B	C	D
6)	A	B	C	D	31)	A	B	C	D	58)	A	B	C	D
7)	A	B	C	D	32)	A	B	C	D	59)	A	B	C	D
8)	A	B	C	D	33)	A	B	C	D	60)	A	B	C	D
9)	A	B	C	D	34)	A	B	C	D	61)	A	B	C	D
10)	A	B	C	D	35)	A	B	C	D	62)	A	B	C	D
11)	A	B	C	D	36)	A	B	C	D	63)	A	B	C	D
12)	A	B	C	D	37)	A	B	C	D	64)	A	B	C	D
13)	A	B	C	D	38)	A	B	C	D	65)	A	B	C	D
14)	A	B	C	D	39)	A	B	C	D	66)	A	B	C	D
15)	A	B	C	D	40)	A	B	C	D	67)	A	B	C	D
16)	A	B	C	D	41)	A	B	C	D	68)	A	B	C	D
17)	A	B	C	D	42)	A	B	C	D	69)	A	B	C	D
18)	A	B	C	D	43)	A	B	C	D	70)	A	B	C	D
19)	A	B	C	D	44)	A	B	C	D	71)	A	B	C	D
20)	A	B	C	D	45)	A	B	C	D	72)	A	B	C	D
21)	A	B	C	D	46)	A	B	C	D	73)	A	B	C	D
22)	A	B	C	D	47)	A	B	C	D	74)	A	B	C	D
23)	A	B	C	D	48)	A	B	C	D	75)	A	B	C	D
24)	A	B	C	D	49)	A	B	C	D	76)	A	B	C	D
25)	A	B	C	D	50)	A	B	C	D	77)	A	B	C	D
					51)	A	B	C	D	78)	A	B	C	D
					52)	A	B	C	D	79)	A	B	C	D

80)	A	B	C	D	107)	A	B	C	D	134)	A	B	C	D
81)	A	B	C	D	108)	A	B	C	D	135)	A	B	C	D
82)	A	B	C	D	109)	A	B	C	D	136)	A	B	C	D
83)	A	B	C	D	110)	A	B	C	D	137)	A	B	C	D
84)	A	B	C	D	111)	A	B	C	D	138)	A	B	C	D
85)	A	B	C	D	112)	A	B	C	D	139)	A	B	C	D
86)	A	B	C	D	113)	A	B	C	D	140)	A	B	C	D
87)	A	B	C	D	114)	A	B	C	D	141)	A	B	C	D
88)	A	B	C	D	115)	A	B	C	D	142)	A	B	C	D
89)	A	B	C	D	116)	A	B	C	D	143)	A	B	C	D
90)	A	B	C	D	117)	A	B	C	D	144)	A	B	C	D
91)	A	B	C	D	118)	A	B	C	D	145)	A	B	C	D
92)	A	B	C	D	119)	A	B	C	D	146)	A	B	C	D
93)	A	B	C	D	120)	A	B	C	D	147)	A	B	C	D
94)	A	B	C	D	121)	A	B	C	D	148)	A	B	C	D
95)	A	B	C	D	122)	A	B	C	D	149)	A	B	C	D
96)	A	B	C	D	123)	A	B	C	D	150)	A	B	C	D
97)	A	B	C	D	124)	A	B	C	D					
98)	A	B	C	D	125)	A	B	C	D					
99)	A	B	C	D	126)	A	B	C	D					
100)	A	B	C	D	127)	A	B	C	D					
101)	A	B	C	D	128)	A	B	C	D					
102)	A	B	C	D	129)	A	B	C	D					
103)	A	B	C	D	130)	A	B	C	D					
104)	A	B	C	D	131)	A	B	C	D					
105)	A	B	C	D	132)	A	B	C	D					
106)	A	B	C	D	133)	A	B	C	D					

Scoring Sheet 10
(tear out for easy use)

#					#					#				
1)	A	B	C	D	26)	A	B	C	D	53)	A	B	C	D
2)	A	B	C	D	27)	A	B	C	D	54)	A	B	C	D
3)	A	B	C	D	28)	A	B	C	D	55)	A	B	C	D
4)	A	B	C	D	29)	A	B	C	D	56)	A	B	C	D
5)	A	B	C	D	30)	A	B	C	D	57)	A	B	C	D
6)	A	B	C	D	31)	A	B	C	D	58)	A	B	C	D
7)	A	B	C	D	32)	A	B	C	D	59)	A	B	C	D
8)	A	B	C	D	33)	A	B	C	D	60)	A	B	C	D
9)	A	B	C	D	34)	A	B	C	D	61)	A	B	C	D
10)	A	B	C	D	35)	A	B	C	D	62)	A	B	C	D
11)	A	B	C	D	36)	A	B	C	D	63)	A	B	C	D
12)	A	B	C	D	37)	A	B	C	D	64)	A	B	C	D
13)	A	B	C	D	38)	A	B	C	D	65)	A	B	C	D
14)	A	B	C	D	39)	A	B	C	D	66)	A	B	C	D
15)	A	B	C	D	40)	A	B	C	D	67)	A	B	C	D
16)	A	B	C	D	41)	A	B	C	D	68)	A	B	C	D
17)	A	B	C	D	42)	A	B	C	D	69)	A	B	C	D
18)	A	B	C	D	43)	A	B	C	D	70)	A	B	C	D
19)	A	B	C	D	44)	A	B	C	D	71)	A	B	C	D
20)	A	B	C	D	45)	A	B	C	D	72)	A	B	C	D
21)	A	B	C	D	46)	A	B	C	D	73)	A	B	C	D
22)	A	B	C	D	47)	A	B	C	D	74)	A	B	C	D
23)	A	B	C	D	48)	A	B	C	D	75)	A	B	C	D
24)	A	B	C	D	49)	A	B	C	D	76)	A	B	C	D
25)	A	B	C	D	50)	A	B	C	D	77)	A	B	C	D
					51)	A	B	C	D	78)	A	B	C	D
					52)	A	B	C	D	79)	A	B	C	D

80)	A	B	C	D	107)	A	B	C	D	134)	A	B	C	D
81)	A	B	C	D	108)	A	B	C	D	135)	A	B	C	D
82)	A	B	C	D	109)	A	B	C	D	136)	A	B	C	D
83)	A	B	C	D	110)	A	B	C	D	137)	A	B	C	D
84)	A	B	C	D	111)	A	B	C	D	138)	A	B	C	D
85)	A	B	C	D	112)	A	B	C	D	139)	A	B	C	D
86)	A	B	C	D	113)	A	B	C	D	140)	A	B	C	D
87)	A	B	C	D	114)	A	B	C	D	141)	A	B	C	D
88)	A	B	C	D	115)	A	B	C	D	142)	A	B	C	D
89)	A	B	C	D	116)	A	B	C	D	143)	A	B	C	D
90)	A	B	C	D	117)	A	B	C	D	144)	A	B	C	D
91)	A	B	C	D	118)	A	B	C	D	145)	A	B	C	D
92)	A	B	C	D	119)	A	B	C	D	146)	A	B	C	D
93)	A	B	C	D	120)	A	B	C	D	147)	A	B	C	D
94)	A	B	C	D	121)	A	B	C	D	148)	A	B	C	D
95)	A	B	C	D	122)	A	B	C	D	149)	A	B	C	D
96)	A	B	C	D	123)	A	B	C	D	150)	A	B	C	D
97)	A	B	C	D	124)	A	B	C	D					
98)	A	B	C	D	125)	A	B	C	D	XXXXXXXXXXXXXX				
99)	A	B	C	D	126)	A	B	C	D	XXXXXXXXXXXXXX				
100)	A	B	C	D	127)	A	B	C	D	XXXXXXXXXXXXXX				
101)	A	B	C	D	128)	A	B	C	D	XXXXXXXXXXXXXX				
102)	A	B	C	D	129)	A	B	C	D					
103)	A	B	C	D	130)	A	B	C	D					
104)	A	B	C	D	131)	A	B	C	D					
105)	A	B	C	D	132)	A	B	C	D					
106)	A	B	C	D	133)	A	B	C	D					

Scoring Sheet 11
(tear out for easy use)

#					#					#				
1)	A	B	C	D	26)	A	B	C	D	53)	A	B	C	D
2)	A	B	C	D	27)	A	B	C	D	54)	A	B	C	D
3)	A	B	C	D	28)	A	B	C	D	55)	A	B	C	D
4)	A	B	C	D	29)	A	B	C	D	56)	A	B	C	D
5)	A	B	C	D	30)	A	B	C	D	57)	A	B	C	D
6)	A	B	C	D	31)	A	B	C	D	58)	A	B	C	D
7)	A	B	C	D	32)	A	B	C	D	59)	A	B	C	D
8)	A	B	C	D	33)	A	B	C	D	60)	A	B	C	D
9)	A	B	C	D	34)	A	B	C	D	61)	A	B	C	D
10)	A	B	C	D	35)	A	B	C	D	62)	A	B	C	D
11)	A	B	C	D	36)	A	B	C	D	63)	A	B	C	D
12)	A	B	C	D	37)	A	B	C	D	64)	A	B	C	D
13)	A	B	C	D	38)	A	B	C	D	65)	A	B	C	D
14)	A	B	C	D	39)	A	B	C	D	66)	A	B	C	D
15)	A	B	C	D	40)	A	B	C	D	67)	A	B	C	D
16)	A	B	C	D	41)	A	B	C	D	68)	A	B	C	D
17)	A	B	C	D	42)	A	B	C	D	69)	A	B	C	D
18)	A	B	C	D	43)	A	B	C	D	70)	A	B	C	D
19)	A	B	C	D	44)	A	B	C	D	71)	A	B	C	D
20)	A	B	C	D	45)	A	B	C	D	72)	A	B	C	D
21)	A	B	C	D	46)	A	B	C	D	73)	A	B	C	D
22)	A	B	C	D	47)	A	B	C	D	74)	A	B	C	D
23)	A	B	C	D	48)	A	B	C	D	75)	A	B	C	D
24)	A	B	C	D	49)	A	B	C	D	76)	A	B	C	D
25)	A	B	C	D	50)	A	B	C	D	77)	A	B	C	D
					51)	A	B	C	D	78)	A	B	C	D
					52)	A	B	C	D	79)	A	B	C	D

PROPERTY OF MEDICAL CODING PRO UNAUTHORIZED DISTRIBUTION PROHIBITED SINGLE COPY LICENSE

80)	A	B	C	D	107)	A	B	C	D	134)	A	B	C	D
81)	A	B	C	D	108)	A	B	C	D	135)	A	B	C	D
82)	A	B	C	D	109)	A	B	C	D	136)	A	B	C	D
83)	A	B	C	D	110)	A	B	C	D	137)	A	B	C	D
84)	A	B	C	D	111)	A	B	C	D	138)	A	B	C	D
85)	A	B	C	D	112)	A	B	C	D	139)	A	B	C	D
86)	A	B	C	D	113)	A	B	C	D	140)	A	B	C	D
87)	A	B	C	D	114)	A	B	C	D	141)	A	B	C	D
88)	A	B	C	D	115)	A	B	C	D	142)	A	B	C	D
89)	A	B	C	D	116)	A	B	C	D	143)	A	B	C	D
90)	A	B	C	D	117)	A	B	C	D	144)	A	B	C	D
91)	A	B	C	D	118)	A	B	C	D	145)	A	B	C	D
92)	A	B	C	D	119)	A	B	C	D	146)	A	B	C	D
93)	A	B	C	D	120)	A	B	C	D	147)	A	B	C	D
94)	A	B	C	D	121)	A	B	C	D	148)	A	B	C	D
95)	A	B	C	D	122)	A	B	C	D	149)	A	B	C	D
96)	A	B	C	D	123)	A	B	C	D	150)	A	B	C	D
97)	A	B	C	D	124)	A	B	C	D					
98)	A	B	C	D	125)	A	B	C	D	XXXXXXXXXXXXXX				
99)	A	B	C	D	126)	A	B	C	D	XXXXXXXXXXXXXX				
100)	A	B	C	D	127)	A	B	C	D	XXXXXXXXXXXXXX				
101)	A	B	C	D	128)	A	B	C	D	XXXXXXXXXXXXXX				
102)	A	B	C	D	129)	A	B	C	D					
103)	A	B	C	D	130)	A	B	C	D					
104)	A	B	C	D	131)	A	B	C	D					
105)	A	B	C	D	132)	A	B	C	D					
106)	A	B	C	D	133)	A	B	C	D					

Scoring Sheet 12
(tear out for easy use)

#					#					#				
1)	A	B	C	D	26)	A	B	C	D	53)	A	B	C	D
2)	A	B	C	D	27)	A	B	C	D	54)	A	B	C	D
3)	A	B	C	D	28)	A	B	C	D	55)	A	B	C	D
4)	A	B	C	D	29)	A	B	C	D	56)	A	B	C	D
5)	A	B	C	D	30)	A	B	C	D	57)	A	B	C	D
6)	A	B	C	D	31)	A	B	C	D	58)	A	B	C	D
7)	A	B	C	D	32)	A	B	C	D	59)	A	B	C	D
8)	A	B	C	D	33)	A	B	C	D	60)	A	B	C	D
9)	A	B	C	D	34)	A	B	C	D	61)	A	B	C	D
10)	A	B	C	D	35)	A	B	C	D	62)	A	B	C	D
11)	A	B	C	D	36)	A	B	C	D	63)	A	B	C	D
12)	A	B	C	D	37)	A	B	C	D	64)	A	B	C	D
13)	A	B	C	D	38)	A	B	C	D	65)	A	B	C	D
14)	A	B	C	D	39)	A	B	C	D	66)	A	B	C	D
15)	A	B	C	D	40)	A	B	C	D	67)	A	B	C	D
16)	A	B	C	D	41)	A	B	C	D	68)	A	B	C	D
17)	A	B	C	D	42)	A	B	C	D	69)	A	B	C	D
18)	A	B	C	D	43)	A	B	C	D	70)	A	B	C	D
19)	A	B	C	D	44)	A	B	C	D	71)	A	B	C	D
20)	A	B	C	D	45)	A	B	C	D	72)	A	B	C	D
21)	A	B	C	D	46)	A	B	C	D	73)	A	B	C	D
22)	A	B	C	D	47)	A	B	C	D	74)	A	B	C	D
23)	A	B	C	D	48)	A	B	C	D	75)	A	B	C	D
24)	A	B	C	D	49)	A	B	C	D	76)	A	B	C	D
25)	A	B	C	D	50)	A	B	C	D	77)	A	B	C	D
					51)	A	B	C	D	78)	A	B	C	D
					52)	A	B	C	D	79)	A	B	C	D

80)	A	B	C	D	107)	A	B	C	D	134)	A	B	C	D
81)	A	B	C	D	108)	A	B	C	D	135)	A	B	C	D
82)	A	B	C	D	109)	A	B	C	D	136)	A	B	C	D
83)	A	B	C	D	110)	A	B	C	D	137)	A	B	C	D
84)	A	B	C	D	111)	A	B	C	D	138)	A	B	C	D
85)	A	B	C	D	112)	A	B	C	D	139)	A	B	C	D
86)	A	B	C	D	113)	A	B	C	D	140)	A	B	C	D
87)	A	B	C	D	114)	A	B	C	D	141)	A	B	C	D
88)	A	B	C	D	115)	A	B	C	D	142)	A	B	C	D
89)	A	B	C	D	116)	A	B	C	D	143)	A	B	C	D
90)	A	B	C	D	117)	A	B	C	D	144)	A	B	C	D
91)	A	B	C	D	118)	A	B	C	D	145)	A	B	C	D
92)	A	B	C	D	119)	A	B	C	D	146)	A	B	C	D
93)	A	B	C	D	120)	A	B	C	D	147)	A	B	C	D
94)	A	B	C	D	121)	A	B	C	D	148)	A	B	C	D
95)	A	B	C	D	122)	A	B	C	D	149)	A	B	C	D
96)	A	B	C	D	123)	A	B	C	D	150)	A	B	C	D
97)	A	B	C	D	124)	A	B	C	D					
98)	A	B	C	D	125)	A	B	C	D	XXXXXXXXXXXXXX				
99)	A	B	C	D	126)	A	B	C	D	XXXXXXXXXXXXXX				
100)	A	B	C	D	127)	A	B	C	D	XXXXXXXXXXXXXX				
101)	A	B	C	D	128)	A	B	C	D	XXXXXXXXXXXXXX				
102)	A	B	C	D	129)	A	B	C	D					
103)	A	B	C	D	130)	A	B	C	D					
104)	A	B	C	D	131)	A	B	C	D					
105)	A	B	C	D	132)	A	B	C	D					
106)	A	B	C	D	133)	A	B	C	D					

Resources

Exam Preparation Products We Recommend

Medical Coding Exam Prep Course
http://medicalcodingpro.com/medical-coding-certification-prep-course

Medical Coding Exam System
http://medicalcodingexamsystem.com

Faster Coder - Code Faster - Code Better
http://fastercoder.com

Other Resources

Elite Members Area – 7 day FREE trial!
http://medicalcodingpromembers.com

Medical Coding Pro – main website
http://medicalcodingpro.com

Code Lookup Program - http://www.findacode.com/?pc=MEDCOPRO

Check out our Checkbook Registers and other log books on Amazon:

https://amzn.to/2NeX1mZ

MEDICAL CODING PRO

Medical Coding Pro provides information about medical coding. We also help people in the medical coding community prepare for the medical coding certification exam.

Our mission is to help everyone we can pass the exam and gain their certification as quickly as possible. To do this we offer quality exam preparation tools such as Medical Coding Practice Exams, the Medical Coding Exam System, the Medical Coding Exam Strategy and the Medical Coding Pro Elite Members Area.

Visit us on the web at:

www.MedicalCodingPro.com

www.MedicalCodingProMembers.com

www.MedicalCodingExamSystem.com

www.MedicalCodingNews.org

CPSIA information can be obtained
at www.ICGtesting.com
Printed in the USA
LVHW021206210820
663295LV00004B/4